Histological Typing of Endocrine Tumours

Springer
Berlin
Heidelberg
New York
Barcelona
Hong Kong
London
Milan
Paris
Singapore
Tokyo

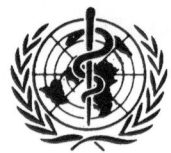 World Health Organization

The series *International Histological Classification of Tumours* consists of the following volumes. The early ones can be ordered through WHO, Distribution and Sales, Avenue Appia, CH-1211 Geneva 27.

A coded compendium of the International Histological Classification of Tumours (1978).

Histological Typing of Endocrine Tumours

E. Solcia G. Klöppel L.H. Sobin

In Collaboration with 9 Pathologists
from 4 Countries

Second Edition

With 122 Colour Figures, 8 Black and White Figures

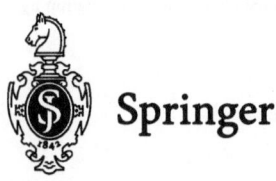 Springer

Enrico Solcia, MD
Department of Pathology
University of Pavia and Policlinico S. Matteo
Via Forlanini 16, 27100 Pavia, Italy

Günter Klöppel, MD
Department of Pathology, University of Kiel
Michaelisstrasse 11, 24105 Kiel, Germany

Leslie H. Sobin, MD
WHO Collaborating Center for the International Histological
Classification of Tumours, Armed Forces Institute of Pathology
Washington, DC 20306-6000, USA

First edition published by WHO in 1980 as No. 23 in the International Histological
Classification of Tumours series.

ISBN-13:978-3-540-66169-6

Library of Congress Cataloging-in-Publication Data
Solcia, Enrico. Histological typing of endocrine tumours / E. Solcia, G. Klöppel, L.H. Sobin; in collaboration with 9 pathologists from 4 countries. - 2nd ed. p. cm. - (International histological classification of tumours) "First edition published by WHO in 1980 as No. 23 in the International histological classification of tumours series." Includes bibliographical references and index.
ISBN-13:978-3-540-66169-6   e-ISBN-13:978-3-642-59655-1
DOI: 10.1007/978-3-642-59655-1

1. Endocrine glands - Tumors - Classification. 2. Endocrine glands - Tumors - Atlases. I. Klöppel, Günter. II. Sobin, L.H. III. Title. IV. International histological classification of tumours (Unnumbered)
RC280.E55.S66 1999   616.99'2407583 - dc21   99-049865

Typesetting: Springer-Verlag, Heidelberg

SPIN: 10730411   24/3135 ih – 5 4 3 2 1 0 – Printed on acid-free paper.

Participants

Capella, C.
Department of Pathology, University of Insubria,
Varese, Italy

DeLellis, R. A.
Department of Pathology, New York Presbyterian Hospital,
New York, NY, USA

Heitz, P. U.
Department of Pathology, University of Zürich,
Zürich, Switzerland

Horvath, E.
Department of Pathology, St. Michael's Hospital,
Toronto, Ontario, Canada

Klöppel, G.
Department of Pathology, University of Kiel,
Kiel, Germany

Kovacs, K.
Department of Pathology, St. Michael's Hospital,
Toronto, Ontario, Canada

Lack, E.
Department of Pathology, Georgetown University School
of Medicine, Washington, DC, USA

Lloyd, R. V.
Department of Laboratory Medicine and Pathology,
Mayo Clinic and Mayo Foundation, Rochester, MN, USA

Rosai, J.
Department of Pathology, Memorial Sloan-Kettering Cancer Center,
New York, NY, USA

Scheithauer, B. W.
Department of Laboratory Medicine and Pathology,
Mayo Clinic and Mayo Foundation, Rochester, MN, USA

Sobin, L.H.
Division of Gastrointestinal Pathology,
Armed Forces Institute of Pathology, Washington, DC, USA

Solcia, E.
Department of Pathology, University of Pavia, Pavia, Italy

General Preface to the Series

Among the prerequisites for comparative studies of cancer are international agreement on histological criteria for the classification of cancer types and a standardized nomenclature. At present, pathologists use different terms for the same pathological entity, and, furthermore, the same term is sometimes applied to lesions of different types. An internationally agreed classification of tumours, acceptable alike to physicians, surgeons, radiologists, pathologists, and statisticians, would enable cancer workers in all parts of the world to compare their findings and would facilitate collaboration among them.

In a report published in 1952[1], a subcommittee of the WHO Expert Committee on Health Statistics discussed the general principles that should govern the statistical classification of tumours and agreed that, to ensure the necessary flexibility and ease in coding, three separate classifications were needed according to (1) anatomical site, (2) histological type, and (3) degree of malignancy. A classification according to anatomical site is available in the International Classification of Diseases[2].

In 1956, the WHO Executive Board passed a resolution[3] requesting the Director-General to explore the possibility that WHO might organise centres in various parts of the world and arrange for the collection of human tissues and their histological classification.

The main purpose of such centres would be to develop histological definitions of cancer types and to facilitate the wide adoption of a uniform nomenclature. This resolution was endorsed by the Tenth World Health Assembly in May, 1957[4].

---

[1] WHO (1952) WHO Technical Report Series, no. 53. WHO, Geneva, p. 45.
[2] WHO (1977) Manual of the international statistical classification of diseases, injuries, and causes of death, 1975 version. WHO, Geneva.
[3] WHO (1956) WHO Official Records, no. 68, p 14 (resolution EB 17.R40).
[4] WHO (1957) WHO Official Records, no. 79, p. 467 (resolution WHA 10.18).

Since 1958, WHO has established a number of centres concerned with this subject. The result of this endeavor has been the International Histological Classification of Tumours, a multivolume series whose first edition was published between 1967 and 1981. The present revised second edition aims to update the classifications, reflecting the progress in diagnosis and relevance of tumour types to clinical and epidemiological features.

Preface to Histological Typing
of Endocrine Tumours – Second Edition

The first edition of *The International Histological Classification of Endocrine Tumours* was published in 1980[1]. Since then, a number of new entities have been recognised, necessitating a revision of the classification.

It will be appreciated, of course, that the classification reflects the present state of knowledge and modifications are almost certain to be needed as experience accumulates. Although the present classification is proposed by the members of the group, it necessarily represents a view to which some pathologists may wish to dissent. Nevertheless, it is hoped that, in the interests of international co-operation, all pathologists will use the classification as proposed. Criticism and suggestions for its improvement will be welcomed – these should be sent to the World Health Organization, 1211 Geneva 27, Switzerland.

The histological classification of endocrine tumours which appears on pp. 7-13, contains the morphology code numbers of the International Classification of Diseases for Oncology (ICD-O)[2] and the Systematised Nomenclature of Medicine (SNOMED)[3].

The publications in the series, International Histological Classification of Tumours, are not intended to serve as textbooks, but rather to promote the adoption of a uniform terminology that will facilitate communication among cancer workers. For this reason, literature references have intentionally been limited; for bibliographies, readers should refer to standard works.

---

[1] Williams ED et al (1980) Histological typing of endocrine tumours. International histological classification of tumours, no. 23. WHO, Geneva
[2] World Health Organization (1990) International classification of diseases for oncology (ICD-O), Geneva.
[3] College of American Pathologists (1982) Systematised nomenclature of medicine (SNOMED), Chicago, IL.

Contents

Introduction

This is a classification of endocrine tumours and tumour-like lesions of the anterior pituitary, adrenal, parathyroid, pancreas, and the diffuse endocrine system. It is based primarily on microscopic characteristics of the tumours, but, where appropriate, it incorporates diagnostically useful immunohistological findings. The most important immunohistological findings helpful in categorising endocrine tumours are summarised in Table 1 (see p.2).

Characterisation of Endocrine Tumours

The histological pattern of most endocrine tumours is characterised by a solid, trabecular, or glandular arrangement of well-differentiated cells which may also form pseudorosettes or tubuloacinar structures. In most cases, these features are sufficiently distinctive to permit recognition of the endocrine nature of the tumour. In other cases, special stains (e.g., silver methods) or immunohistochemical stains for general neuroendocrine markers (e.g., chromogranins, synaptophysin, or neuron-specific enolase) are needed for tumour identification. In addition, immunohistochemical stains for hormones and, occasionally, electron microscopy are necessary to characterise tumour cell types and their specific hormonal products, which may cause a syndrome of endocrine hyperfunction correlating to the biological behaviour of the tumour. Hence, there is a need to integrate histology and hormonally characterised cell types into a so-called "morphofunctional" classification.

When carefully investigated, many tumours prove to be composed of more than one cell type. Sometimes they are composed of several cell types. As a rule, only one of them correlates to an associated syndrome of endocrine hyperfunction. For this reason, classifying endocrine tumours by cell-typing alone is of limited value in

Table 1. Differential immunohistology of common endocrine tumours (ET)

Site and tumour type	CK8,18	VIM	CEA	S-100	SYN	CG	Principal hormones
Pituitary adenoma	±	-	-	-[a]	+	±	PRL,GH,ACTH,TSH,FSH,LH
Parathyroid adenoma	+	-	-	-	+	+	Parathyroid hormone
Thyroid medullary carcinoma	+	-	+	-[a]	+	+	Calcitonin
Lung ET	+	-	-	-	+	+	Bombesin, serotonin, calcitonin
Thymic ET	+	-	-	-	+	+	ACTH
Gastric ET	+	-	-	-	+	+	Histamine, serotonin
Duodenal ET	+	-	-[a]	-	+	+	Gastrin, somatostatin, serotonin
Ileal ET	+	-	-	-[a]	+	+	Serotonin, substance P
Appendiceal ET	+	-	-	-[a]	+	+	Serotonin, substance P
Colorectal ET	+	-	-	-	+	+	Enteroglucagon, PP/PYY; serotonin, substance P
Pancreatic ET	+	-	-	-	+	+	Insulin, gastrin, glucagon, VIP, somatostatin, PP
Paraganglioma, head/neck	-[a]	+[c]	-	+[b]	+	+	Serotonin, dopamine, noradrenalin
Paraganglioma, sympathetic	-[a]	+[c]	-	+[b]	+	+	Noradrenalin, dopamine
Pheochromocytoma	-[a]	+[c]	-	+[b]	+	+	Adrenalin, noradrenalin
Adrenal cortex tumour	+	-[a]	-	-	+[d]	-	Steroid hormones

[a] Positivity in rare tumours. [b] Positivity in sustentacular cells. [c] Positivity in sustentacular cells and endothelial cells.
[d] Positivity in up to 80% of tumours.
CK, cytokeratin; VIM, vimentin; CEA, carcinoembryonic antigen; S-100, S-100 protein; SYN, synaptophysin; CG, chromogranin; PRL, prolactin; GH, growth hormone; ACTH, adrenocorticotropic hormone; TSH, thyroid-stimulating hormone; FSH, follicle-stimulating hormone; LH, luteinising hormone; PP, pancreatic polypeptide; PYY, peptide with N-terminal and C-terminal tyrosine; VIP, vasoactive intestinal peptide.

practice unless correlated to clinical signs and symptoms, and hormonal measurements in the blood. It is known that some tumours, especially in the pituitary and pancreas, are frequently associated with a range of well-defined hyperfunctional syndromes which determine the clinicopathological profile of the disease and are usually more predictive of the tumour's natural history than purely morphological findings. In such cases, the tumour itself may be designated according to the associated hyperfunctional syndrome, for example, as "insulinoma" or "gastrinoma", etc. Such syndrome-based labeling

Table 2. General endocrine tumour categories

1	Well-differentiated endocrine tumour
2	Well-differentiated endocrine carcinoma
3	Poorly differentiated endocrine (small cell) carcinoma
4	Mixed exocrine-endocrine tumour
5	Tumour-like lesions

should not be used to designate clinically nonfunctioning (nonsyndromic) tumours lacking an associated hyperfunctional syndrome, even when hormones are detected in tumour cells and/or the serum. Such hormonal contents should be mentioned in the report (e.g., "pancreatic endocrine tumour, glucagon-producing") as a basis for further clinicopathological and follow-up investigations.

The need for a close correlation between morphological classification and associated endocrine syndromes is underscored by the difficulty in predicting the biological behaviour of well-differentiated endocrine tumours when using classical histopathological malignancy criteria (e.g., cellular or structural atypia, necrosis, mitotic activity, or microscopic invasion). Moreover, available follow-up studies refer mostly to tumours diagnosed according to the associated syndrome. For these reasons, clinicopathological correlations are given in the explanatory notes and outlined on tables.

In general, three main categories of tumours have been recognised: 1) well-differentiated endocrine tumours, 2) poorly differentiated endocrine carcinomas, and 3) mixed exocrine-endocrine tumours (Table 2). The basis for distinguishing low-grade endocrine carcinomas from other well-differentiated endocrine tumours is usually the presence of metastases and/or evidence of local invasion. Benign (or low risk) endocrine tumours are distinguished from tumours with a greater risk of malignancy on the basis of a combination of features such as tumour size and site, local extension, angioinvasion, cellular atypia, mitotic index/proliferative activity, and tissue-appropriate (eutopic) or -inappropriate (ectopic) hormonal products in conjunction with endocrine syndromes. Distinguishing poorly differentiated endocrine small cell carcinoma from well-differentiated endocrine neoplasms is easy in conventional histological preparations, given the distinctive pattern of the former tumour, which shows high-grade cellular atypia with markedly hyperchromatic nuclei, a high nuclear/cytoplasmic ratio with poorly defined borders, high mitotic/proliferative indices, and focal necrosis. As a rule, this tumour shows diffuse reactivity for cytosolic neuroendocrine markers such as, synaptophysin neuron-specific enolase (NSE) or protein gene product (PGP) 9.5. In contrast, reactivity with markers of endocrine granules such as chromogranins or Grimelius silver, is scant to weak; and immunostaining for hormonal or neurosecretory products is poor to absent. Occasionally, some endocrine tumours may show both well-differentiated and poorly differentiated components, suggesting a possible evolution of one type into the other. However, in most cases, small cell endocrine carcinoma seems to arise independently of other preceding or associated tumour types.

A few moderately differentiated tumours with cellular and structural atypia intermediate between those of well and poorly differentiated tumours have been observed. Among the distinctive features of such tumours are large, solid cellular aggregates and large trabeculae with crowding and irregular distribution of hyperchromatic or vesicular nuclei with prominent nucleoli and irregular chromatin clumps, considerable mitotic activity, sometimes with atypical mitotic figures and scant necrosis, combined with substantial, widespread reactivity for endocrine markers, both granular and cytosolic. Tumours showing this histological pattern have been reported in the lung (see the pertinent publication in this series) under the term "atypical carcinoids". Their clinical behaviour has been found to be more aggressive than that of usual nonatypical carcinoids (i.e., well-differentiated endocrine tumours), though less aggressive than that of small cell (or poorly differentiated) endocrine carcinomas. Although there is some evidence that similar neoplasms may also arise in the gut and the pancreas, this still seems insufficient cause to introduce a separate category at these sites or, for that matter, in the general classification of endocrine tumours. Nevertheless, while waiting for elucidation of this issue, it would seem advisable to mention such "atypical" or moderately differentiated patterns in histological reports. In tumours lacking clinical evidence of malignancy (metastases, local invasion, etc), this may warn the physician of increased risk and stimulate additional investigations and closer follow-up. In malignant tumours, this pattern may be a forerunner of more aggressive behaviour or result in shorter survival rates and/or the need for a more aggressive therapy.

With regard to mixed tumours, only those showing quantitatively balanced amounts of endocrine and exocrine components, whether within the same cell (amphicrine) as separate but intimately admixed cells (combined tumours) or as separate tumour growths (composite tumours), should be classified as mixed exocrine-endocrine tumours. Tumours that are primarily exocrine but show a minority of dispersed endocrine cells (which are unlikely to influence their behaviour) are not to be considered in the context of the present classification.

The term "tumour" is used synonymously with "neoplasm". The phrase "tumour-like" is applied to lesions that clinically or morphologically resemble neoplasms but do not behave biologically as true neoplasms. Tumour-like lesions are included in this classification because of their importance in the differential diagnosis and because, in some cases, the borderline between true neoplasms and certain non-neoplastic lesions remains unclear.

The classification shown in Table 2 applies both to tumours arising in primarily endocrine structures, such as pituitary, adrenals, and parathyroids, and to tumours arising in structures with only a limited endocrine component, such as pancreas, gastrointestinal mucosa, lung, prostate, ovary, testes, and skin. In addition, it covers endocrine tumours arising in tissues which, in humans, are normally devoid of a significant endocrine component, such as thymus, oesophagus, larynx, biliary tract, liver, kidney, or uterus. Here, we shall only deal with tumours of the pituitary, adrenals, parathyroids, pancreas, and gastrointestinal tract. For endocrine or mixed endocrine/exocrine tumours arising in other sites, the reader is referred to the pertinent publication in the series.

Histological Classification
of Endocrine Tumours

1 Histological Classification
of Adenohypophyseal Tumours

1.1   Adenoma
1.1.1 *Typical* .... *8272/0*[1,2]
1.1.2 *Atypical* *8272/1*

1.2   Carcinoma *8272/3*

1.3   Soft Tissue Tumours
1.3.1 *Post-irradiation sarcoma*
1.3.2 *Benign soft tissue tumours*

1.4   Secondary tumours

1.5   Tumour-like lesions
1.5.1 *Pituitary hyperplasia*
1.5.2 *Rathke cleft cyst*
1.5.3 *Lymphocytic hypophysitis*
1.5.4 *Giant cell granuloma*

---

[1] Morphology code of the International Classification of Diseases for Oncology (ICD-O) and the Systematized Nomenclature of Medicine (SNOMED). Behaviour is coded /0 for benign tumours, /3 for malignant tumours, and /1 for unspecified, borderline or uncertain behaviour.

[2] The italicized numbers are provisional codes proposed for the third edition of ICD-O. They should, for the most part, be incorporated into the next edition of ICD-O, but they are subject to change.

2   Histological Classification of Tumours of the Adrenal Cortex

3   Histological Classification of Tumours of Adrenal and Extra-adrenal Paraganglia

4   Histological Classification of Tumours of the Parathyroid Glands

5   Histological Classification of Endocrine Tumours of the Pancreas

6   Histological Classification of Endocrine Tumours of the Gastrointestinal Tract

6.1.5   *Tumour-like lesions*
6.1.5.1   Hyperplasia
6.1.5.2   Dysplasia (precarcinoid lesions)

**6.2   Histological Classification of Endocrine Tumours
of the Duodenum and Upper Jejunum**
6.2.1   *Well-differentiated endocrine tumour – carcinoid*   8240/1
6.2.1.1   Gastrin-producing tumour, functioning (gastrinoma)
or nonfunctioning 8153/1
6.2.1.2   Somatostatin-producing tumour *8156/1*
6.2.1.3   Serotonin-producing tumour, nonfunctioning ..   8241/1
6.2.1.4   Gangliocytic paraganglioma 8683/0
6.2.1.5   Others
6.2.2   *Well-differentiated endocrine carcinoma –
malignant carcinoid* 8240/3
6.2.2.1   Gastrin-producing carcinoma, mostly functioning
(gastrinoma) 8153/3
6.2.2.2   Somatostatin-producing carcinoma *8156/3*
6.2.2.3   Serotonin-producing carcinoma, functioning
or nonfunctioning 8241/3
6.2.2.4   Malignant gangliocytic paraganglioma 8683/3
6.2.2.5   Others
6.2.3   *Poorly differentiated endocrine carcinoma –
small cell carcinoma* 8041/3

**6.3   Histological Classification of Endocrine Tumours
of the Ileum, Caecum, Colon, and Rectum**
6.3.1   *Well-differentiated endocrine tumour – carcinoid*   8240/1
6.3.1.1   Serotonin-producing tumour 8241/1
6.3.1.2   Enteroglucagon-producing tumour *8157/1*
6.3.1.3   Others
6.3.2   *Well differentiated endocrine carcinoma –
malignant carcinoid* 8240/3
6.3.2.1   Serotonin-producing carcinoid with or without
carcinoid syndrome 8241/3
6.3.2.2   Enteroglucagon-producing carcinoma *8157/3*
6.3.3   *Poorly differentiated endocrine carcinoma –
small cell carcinoma* 8041/3
6.3.4   *Mixed exocrine-endocrine carcinoma* 8244/3

Definitions and Explanatory Notes

1   Tumours of the Adenohypophysis

Adenohypophyseal tumours, almost all of which are adenomas, have been variously classified on the basis of their clinical presentation, biochemical findings, histology (growth pattern and tinctorial characteristics), proliferation activity, immunocytochemical profile, and ultrastructural features. Herein, we propose a five-tier classification, clinicopathological in nature, which focuses not only upon histology, immunocytochemistry (Table 3, p. 20), ultrastructure (Table 4, p. 22), but endocrine activity (Table 5, p. 26) and imaging, as well as operative findings (Table 6, p. 28). In the case of pituitary tumours, integration of these five complementary approaches to what is fundamentally a pathological classification is practical. It provides valuable information to clinical endocrinologists, neurosurgeons, and oncologists involved in the assessment of a tumour's biological behaviour, growth potential, therapeutic responsiveness, and prognosis. Due to financial constraints, lack of facilities, and unavailability of well-trained personnel, it is recognised that the five approaches cannot be fully implemented worldwide. Nonetheless, in addition to basic histological parameters, clinical and biochemical data as well as imaging and operative findings are generally readily available. Collectively, they are indispensable in establishing a correct diagnosis and in directing patient management. Clearly, consideration of endocrine activity and growth characteristics in addition to histological, immunophenotypic, and ultrastructural features provides greater insight into the pathobiology of adenohypophyseal tumours than does routine histology alone. Thus, the inclusion of immunocytochemical and ultrastructural investigation into a modern classification is fully justified.

1.1   Adenoma (Figs. 1, 2, 4–15)

1.1.1   Typical Adenoma

A histologically benign neoplasm of adenohypophyseal cells.

Adenomas exhibit a variety of relatively nonspecific histological patterns, e.g., diffuse, sinusoidal, pseudorosette, and papillary. Although these are not considered to be important to classification, certain patterns do suggest specific functional differentiation. For example, tumours with perivascular pseudorosette or papilla formation are often glycoprotein hormone-producing. Other correlations of morphology with differentiation include a) the formation of calcospherites or spherical amyloid bodies in prolactin cell adenomas, b) the formation of cytoplasmic fibrous bodies in GH cell adenomas of sparsely granulated (chromophobic) type, and c) Crooke hyalinisation, a cytoplasmic alteration generally limited to nontumoural ACTH cells in the setting of Cushing syndrome, ectopic ACTH/CRH syndrome, or glucocorticoid excess of exogenous type. Widespread Crooke hyalinisation is rarely a feature of ACTH adenoma cells (Crooke cell adenoma).

Tinctorial characteristics are no longer the basis of adenoma classification. Nonetheless, assessment of optimal H&E and PAS-stained sections may provide insight into the nature of the hormone(s) produced. For example, strongly acidophilic tumours are often GH-producing, whereas ampho- or basophilic PAS-positive adenomas are typically ACTH-producing. Lack of staining, as in chromophobic adenomas, does not signify lack of hormone production or endocrine activity.

The large majority of pituitary adenomas are "typical", being monomorphic proliferations composed of cells with uniform round nuclei, delicate stippled chromatin, inconspicuous nucleoli, and moderate quantities of cytoplasm. As a rule, mitoses are rare or lacking entirely. Ki 67 (MIB-1 antibody) labeling indices are generally in the range of 0–3% for noninvasive adenomas. It is of note that cellular pleomorphism, nuclear abnormalities, cellularity, haemorrhage, and necrosis are not reliable indicators of aggressive behaviour. All adenohypophyseal tumours may be described in terms of their size as micro- or macroadenomas, i.e. tumours up to or greater than 1 cm in maximal dimension.

1.1.2.   Atypical Adenoma (Fig. 2)

An adenoma with atypical morphologic features suggestive of aggressive behaviour.

Aggressive behaviour refers to invasive growth and implies the potential for recurrence.The main atypical morphological feature is an elevated mitotic index, mitototic figures being more than scant. An MIB-1 labeling index greater than 3 percent, is another.

It is also of note that 15% of invasive adenomas have been found to express p53 immunoreactivity, a feature generally lacking in noninvasive adenomas seen in approximately 15% of invasive tumours, and present in nearly all pituitary carcinomas. The designation "atypical" is not based upon tumour invasiveness. Typical adenomas may be invasive of pituitary parenchyma, the dural envelope surrounding the gland, or nearby bone and soft tissue. The two major growth patterns include:
a) Expansive. Radiographically or grossly apparent, this pattern features a demarcated, compressive tumour interface with surrounding tissue.
b) Invasive (bone, nerve, vessels, etc). This feature is radiographically or grossly defined, since, as previously stated, microscopic dural invasion is common in typical microadenomas and increases in frequency with tumour size. Microscopic dural invasion is, therefore, not considered a reliable indicator of aggressive tumour behaviour.

1.2   Pituitary Carcinoma (Fig. 3)

A tumour of adenohypophyseal cells showing metastasis and/or brain invasion.

Malignancy in adenohypophyseal tumours is manifested either as craniospinal or systemic metastases, or as brain invasion. Such tumours vary considerably in their histological and cytological appearance. Whereas some resemble ordinary pituitary adenomas, most show increased mitotic activity, a significantly increased MIB-1 labeling index, and p53 immunoreactivity.

1.3   Soft Tissue Tumours

Aside from pituitary adenoma and the occasional carcinoma, primary soft tissue tumours arising in the adenohypophysis are exceedingly rare. Best-known are postirradiation sarcomas, usually fibrosarcoma or osteosarcoma. Benign tumours include hemangioma, glomangioma, and fibroma. The histological distinction of these lesions from tumours of adenohypophyseal cells generally poses no diagnostic problem.

1.3.1   Postirradiation Sarcoma

1.3.2   Benign Soft Tissue Tumours

1.4   Secondary Tumours

Secondary tumours rarely affect the adenohypophysis directly. Instead, most represent extension from neurohypophyseal or bony sellar deposits. Although relatively common in autopsy series, involvement of the adenohypophysis infrequently manifests clinically and is rarely the presenting sign of a malignant neoplasm. Common sources include carcinoma of breast and lung. Haematolymphoid tumours include leukaemia, lymphoma, and plasmacytoma. Sarcomas, usually fibro- or osteosarcomas, are usually a complication of prior irradiation to the sellar region.

1.5   Tumour-like Lesions

1.5.1   Pituitary Hyperplasia (Fig. 16)

The lesion ranges from a) a mild, diffuse increase in number of a specific cell type not causing significant distortion of the normal acinar architecture to b) massive nodular hyperplasia resulting in marked distension and limited confluence of acini, as well as to enlargement of the entire gland. This rare process poses a significant diagnostic challenge and is usually associated with overt signs and symptoms of endocrine dysfunction. Due to the normally uneven distribution of most pituitary cell types and the fragmented nature of surgical specimens, diffuse hyperplasia is difficult, if not impossible, to diagnose in a surgical specimen. Of particular clinical importance are:

a) ACTH cell hyperplasia necessitating total hypophysectomy for cure of Cushing syndrome,
b) TSH cell hyperplasia which may mimic adenoma, but in most cases does not require surgical intervention, since it is often amenable to thyroid hormone replacement,
c) GH cell hyperplasia occurring primarily in association with ectopic growth hormone-releasing hormone (GRH) production by neuroendocrine neoplasms,
d) PRL cell hyperplasia, the result of "pituitary stalk section effect" due to neoplastic or non-neoplastic processes in the suprasellar region or of oestrogen administration, etc. Idiopathic PRL cell hyperplasia is exceptionally rare and of no clinical significance. PRL cell hyperplasia is a regular feature of pregnancy.
    FSH/LH cell hyperplasia, although a prominent feature in Klinefelter and Turner syndrome, has yet to be described in surgical material.

1.5.2   Rathke Cleft Cyst

An intra- or suprasellar, unilocular cyst composed of a single layer of mucin-secreting and/or ciliated columnar to cuboidal epithelial cells.

Stroma is scant. Metaplastic and degenerative changes are common and include squamous metaplasia and xanthogranulomatous change.

1.5.3   Lymphocytic Hypophysitis

A diffuse adenohypophyseal infiltrate composed of mature lymphocytes and, to a lesser extent, plasma cells.

As a rule, macrophages are scant and no granulomas are noted. Chronic lesions feature interstitial fibrosis. Microbiological studies are negative for organisms. There is a strong female predilection and association with pregnancy.

1.5.4   Giant Cell Granuloma

A non-necrotizing granulomatous lesion of the adenohypophysis composed of epithelioid macrophages and multinucleate giant cells.

Schaumann bodies may be seen ultrastructural studies reveal no Birbeck granules. Microbiological studies are negative for organisms.

Immunohistochemical Features of Adenohypophysial Tumours
(Table 3, Figs. 4–15)

Whereas synaptophysin and neuron-specific enolase immunoreactivity is common to pituitary adenomas of all types, chromogranin staining is primarily a feature of glycoprotein hormone (LH, FSH, TSH, and alpha subunit)-producing adenomas, plurihormonal tumours, and null cell adenomas. Although the demonstration of specific hormones in adenomas permits their classification, the hormonal immunophenotype of endocrinologically functioning adenomas is often more complex than the clinical picture suggests. This is particularly the case in growth-hormone-producing adenomas among which plurihormonal examples are the rule, the most frequent phenotypes being GH, PRL, TSH, and alpha subunit. We therefore refer to principal (clinically relevant) and secondary immunoreactivities. By convention and due to structural homology of the hormones, tumours producing GH and PRL as well as LH and FSH, are not considered plurihormonal.

Table 3. Immunohistochemical classification of adenohypophyseal tumours

Principal immunoreactivity	Secondary immunoreactivity[a]
A. GH	PRL, α-SU(f), TSH, FSH, LH(i)
B. PRL	α-SU(i)
C. GH and PRL	α-SU(f), TSH(i)
D. ACTH	LH, α-SU(i)
E. TSH	α-SU(f), GH, PRL(i)
F. FSH/LH/aSU	PRL, GH, ACTH(i)
G. Plurihormonal[b]	
H. Hormone immunonegative	

[a] Secondary hormone immunoreactivities are commonly observed. Although most are not clinically expressed, the hormones may be biochemically detected in blood.
[b] Combinations of immunoreactivities, the most common being GH/PRL/TSH and/or aSU. Other combinations are rare, e.g., ACTH-LH, GH-ACTH, PRL-TSH, etc.
GH, growth hormone; PRL, prolactin; ACTH, adrenocorticotropic hormone; LH, luteinising hormone; FSH, follicle-stimulating hormone; TSH, thyrotropin; a-SU, alpha subunit; i, infrequent; f, frequent

Since normal, nontumourous adenohypophysis is often over-run, its cells becoming incorporated within the substance of an adenoma, it may be impossible to decide whether minor immunoreactivities represent neoplastic or intermingled normal cells. Careless study thus artificially raises the incidence of plurihormonality in pituitary adenomas. A critical approach mindful of frequently occurring hormone combinations is necessary in the interpretation of immunostains.

Morphological Features of Adenohypophysial Tumour Types and Variants (Tables 3, 4)

Growth Hormone Cell Adenoma (Fig. 17)

Densely granulated (DG-GH)
- Centrally situated nuclei, relatively lucent cytoplasm, numerous, uniformly electron-dense, spherical, predominantly 300–500 nm secretory granules. Granules >600 nm may be ovoid or irregular. Tubuloreticular aggregates may be seen in the perinuclear cisterns of epithelial cells.
- Utility of ultrastructure: optional if GH immunoreactivity is convincing; usually slow-growing.

Sparsely granulated (SG-GH)
- Variable cell size. Eccentric, flattened, or crescent-shaped nucleus indented by spherical fibrous body composed of intermediate (cytokeratin) filaments, smooth endoplasmic reticulum, and entrapped organelles, including centrioles. Sparse, small (up to 250 nm), randomly scattered secretory granules. Tubuloreticular aggregates (see above) may be present.
- Utility of ultrastructure: optional if GH immunoreactivity is convincing and cytokeratin antisera detect juxtanuclear fibrous bodies; likely to be aggressive.

Prolactin Cell Adenoma (Fig. 18)

Sparsely granulated (SG-PRL)
- Masses of rough endoplasmic reticulum (RER) organised in parallel cisternae or concentric whorls. Prominent Golgi complex containing spherical and pleomorphic, maturing granules; sparse, up to 300 nm secretory granules. Extrusion of secretory granules,

Table 4. Ultrastructural classification of adenohypophyseal tumours

Tumour type	Variant
Growth hormone cell adenoma	Densely granulated
	Sparsely granulated
Prolactin cell adenoma	Densely granulated
	Sparsely granulated
Adenomas with growth hormone and prolactin cell differentiation	Mixed GH-PRL cell adenoma
	Mammosomatotroph cell adenoma
	Acidophil stem cell adenoma
ACTH cell adenoma	Densely granulated
	Sparsely granulated
	Crooke cell variant
TSH cell adenoma	
FSH-LH cell adenoma	Male type
	Female type
Null cell adenoma	Non-oncocytic
	Oncocytic
Other adenomas	Silent "corticotroph" subtype 1
	Silent "corticotroph" subtype 2
	Silent adenoma subtype 3
	Plurimorphous adenomas,e.g., GH-PRL-TSH, PRL-ACTH, etc.
	Unclassified

singly or grouped, at other than the vascular interface ("misplaced exocytosis").
- Utility of ultrastructure: optional, if Golgi-pattern PRL immunoreactivity is strong and generalised. Slightly to moderately elevated serum PRL and scanty or inconclusive tissue PRL immunoreactivity calls for EM confirmation of diagnosis.

Densely granulated (DG-PRL)
- Less prominent RER. Numerous spherical and irregular, up to 600 nm secretory granules engaged in "misplaced exocytosis" (see above). Extruding granules may have an uneven, blotchy texture.
- Utility of ultrastructure: optional if PRL immunoreactivity is strong. Very rare variant of no clinical relevance.

Adenomas with Growth Hormone and Prolactin Cell Differentiation
(Figs. 18, 19)

Mixed GH cell-PRL cell
- Bimorphous mixture of SG-PRL and DG-GH (or rarely SG-GH) cells.

Mammosomatotroph cell
- Similar to DG-GH, but granule size tends to be larger (up to 1000 nm). Irregular secretory granules with rarefied, mottled texture. Misplaced granule exocytosis is often seen.

Acidophil stem cell (ASCA)
- Oncocytic change with formation of giant mitochondria, aggregates of smooth endoplasmic reticulum, and/or fibrous body formation (infrequent). Granule extrusion (frequently orthotopic) of the often scant, small secretory granules (<250 nm) is frequently seen.
- Utility of ultrastructure: mandatory for separation of mixed GH-PRL cell adenoma due to overlapping immunohistochemical profiles. Mammosomatotroph cell adenoma is slow-growing, whereas mixed GH-PRL cell and acidophil stem cell adenoma may be aggressive.

ACTH Cell Adenoma (Figs. 20,21)

Densely granulated ACTH (DG-ACTH)
- Relatively electron-dense cytoplasm. Numerous, variably electron-dense, spherical to indented, drop- or heart-shaped secretory granules, most measuring 300–450 nm; bundles of intermediate (cytokeratin) filaments.
- Utility of ultrastructure: optional if the basophilic tumour is convincingly immunoreactive for ACTH; usually microadenoma.

Sparsely granulated ACTH (SG-ACTH)
- Secretory granules less characteristic in morphology than in DG-ACTH adenomas, being more spherical, smaller (150–300 nm) and peripherally located beneath the plasma membrane. Intermediate filament (cytokeratin) bundles are scant.
- Utility of ultrastructure: may be necessary if ACTH immunoreactivity is scant or inconclusive; it is likely to be an aggressive macroadenoma.

Crooke cell adenoma
- Similar to DG-ACTH adenoma, but features massive perinuclear, ring-like accumulation of intermediate (cytokeratin) filaments. Secretory granules are displaced to the cell periphery and entrapped within the Golgi region.
- Utility of ultrastructure: optional, if ACTH immunoreactivity is conclusive; morphological variant with no obvious clinical relevance.

Thyrotroph Cell Adenoma (Fig. 21)

TSH Cell
- Variable cell size and morphology. Cells are often polar with small (up to 250 nm), peripherally disposed secretory granules. Some nuclear pleomorphism and perivascular as well as interstitial fibrosis may be seen.
- Utility of ultrastructure: mandatory for diagnosis if clinical presentation and TSH immunoreactivity are not convincing.

Gonadotroph Cell Adenoma (Fig. 22)

FSH/LH Cell, Male Type
- Polar attenuated cells, variable RER, sparse, small (up to 200 nm) subplasmalemmal secretory granules accumulated in cell processes. Oncocytic change and follicle formation are common. Cytoplasmic "light bodies" similar in size to mitochondria and bounded by a single-ruffled membrane may be seen.

FSH/LH Cell, Female Type
- Same as above with the exception of the marker of the variant, the vesicular transformation of Golgi apparatus ("honeycomb Golgi"). Light bodies (see above) and follicle formation may be seen.
- Utility of ultrastructure: mandatory for identification of tumour types but not essential for clinical management, since FSH-LH and null cell tumours have overlapping immunohistochemical profiles and similar biological behaviour.

Null Cell Adenoma (Fig. 23)

Nononcocytic

Small, polyhedral cells with poorly developed RER and Golgi membranes and small (200 nm), sparse, variably dense secretory granules.

Oncocytic

Larger cells with same features as nononcocytic null cell but with the addition of mitochondrial abundance.

- Utility of ultrastructure: mandatory for identification of tumour types but not essential for clinical management, since FSH-LH and null cell tumours have overlapping immunohistochemical profiles and similar biological behaviour.

Other Adenomas (Fig. 24)

Silent "corticotroph" cell adenoma, subtype 1

- Indistinguishable from endocrinologically active DG-ACTH cell adenoma.
- Utility of ultrastructure: optional if basophilia, ACTH immunoreactivity, and lack of Cushing syndrome are established.

Silent "corticotroph" cell adenoma, subtype 2

- Slightly smaller than average, polyhedral cells with unremarkable RER and Golgi membranes, varying numbers of small to middle size (200–400 nm), slightly irregular, and often drop-shaped secretory granules. Microfilament bundles are lacking.
- Utility of ultrastructure: mandatory for recognition of this tumour type.

Silent adenoma, subtype 3

- Large, slightly polar cells; often irregular nuclei containing spherical nuclear inclusions (spheridia); abundant RER, and frequently SER; extensive, tortuous Golgi complex; variable number of spherical, approximately 200 nm secretory granules. Multiple foci of cell membrane interdigitation.
- Utility of ultrastructure: mandatory for diagnosis, which is essential for appropriate management.

Plurimorphous adenomas
- Most are composed of DG-GH and of TSH cells, other combinations being rare. Such tumours correspond to the plurihormonal immunotype.
- Utility of ultrastructure: highly advisable to characterise phenotype(s).

Unclassified Adenomas
- Adenomas composed of often unique cells lacking specific morphological markers.
- Utility of ultrastructure: highly advisable to characterise phenotype(s).

Functional Features of Adenohypophyseal Tumours (Table 5)

1. Endocrine hyperfunction. Hyperfunction can be manifest either clinically or biochemically by serum hormone level elevation(s).
   a) Acromegaly/gigantism; elevated serum GH levels.
   b) Hyperprolactinaemia and sequelae. Serum prolactin elevations less than fourfold normally do not necessarily signify tumoural prolactin production. Instead, it may be due to compression of the pituitary stalk with interruption of the delivery of dopamine, the physiological prolactin inhibiting factor

Table 5. Functional classification of adenohypophyseal tumours

1	Endocrine hyperfunction,
1.1	Acromegaly/gigantism, elevated growth hormone levels
1.2	Hyperprolactinaemia and sequelae
1.3	Cushing syndrome, elevated ACTH and cortisol levels
1.4	Hyperthyroidism with inappropriate secretion of TSH
1.5	Significantly elevated FSH/LH and/or alpha subunit levels
1.6	Multiple hormonal overproduction
2	Clinically nonfunctioning
3	Functional status undetermined
4	Endocrine hyperfunction due to ectopic sources
4.1	Clinical acromegaly secondary to ectopic GRH overproduction
4.2	Cushing syndrome secondary to ectopic CRH overproduction

ACTH, adrenocorticotropic hormone; TSH, thyrotroph-stimulating hormone; FSH, follicle-stimulating hormone; LH, luteinising hormone; GRH, growth-hormone-releasing hormone; CRH, corticotropin-releasing hormone.

(PIF), to normal prolactin cells of the pituitary. The result of this "stalk section effect" is to permit excess prolactin secretion. Stress and endocrine abnormalities, such as oestrogen administration or TRH elevation, may also stimulate excess prolactin production.

  c) Cushing syndrome; elevated serum ACTH and cortisol levels.
  d) Hyperthyroidism with inappropriate secretion of TSH.
  e) Significantly elevated FSH/LH and/or alpha subunit levels.
  f) Multiple hormone overproduction. This can result from the activity of a single plurihormonal adenoma or, on occasion, the presence of multiple functioning adenomas.

2. Clinically nonfunctioning. This includes situations wherein a) no known hormone is produced or released, as in the case of null cell adenomas, b) hormones or hormone fragments are produced which generally do not cause clinical manifestations, e.g., FSH, LH, and alpha subunit, c) a hormone normally causing manifestations is produced, e.g., ACTH and GH, but without clinical or biochemical evidence of its secretion, and d) a biologically inactive hormone fragment or a prohormone is produced.

3. Functional status undetermined.

4. Endocrine hyperfunction due to ectopic sources. Endocrine hyperfunction due to ectopic sources include a) the production of hypothalamic-releasing hormones by a variety of neoplasms, mostly neuroendocrine in nature, and b) the production of pituitary hormones by extrapituitary tumours. Pituitary changes include hyperplasia with or without adenoma.

Imaging and Surgical Features of Adenohypophyseal Tumours
(Table 6)

Location

1. Intrasellar. Many pituitary adenomas are limited to the sella which accommodates their volume by expansion and bony remodeling. Marked sellar expansion may result in virtual loss of the bony sella without actual bone invasion.

2. Extrasellar extension. Extrasellar extension occurs in various directions, including a) suprasellar extension, wherein the sellar diaphragm is elevated or, being incomplete, poses no barrier to upward tumour growth, b) extension into the sphenoid sinus or

Table 6. Imaging/surgical classification of adenohypophyseal tumours

1	Location
1.1	Intrasellar
1.2	Extrasellar extension
	(suprasellar, sphenoid sinus, nasopharynx, cavernous sinus, etc.)
1.3	Ectopic (rare)
2	Size
2.1	Microadenoma ($\leq$10 mm)
2.2	Macroadenoma (>10 mm)
3	Growth pattern
3.1	Expansive
3.2	Grossly invasive of dura, bone, nerves, or brain
3.3	Metastasising (craniospinal or systemic); rare

nasopharynx after extensive erosion of the bony sella has taken place, or c) cavernous sinus extension, which results from lateral tumour growth with either displacement of the thin dural membrane separating the sella from the sinus, or growth through naturally occurring defects in the membrane.

3. Ectopic. Rare examples of ectopic pituitary adenomas usually lie in the suprasellar region but may occur within the sphenoid or ethmoid sinus.

Size

1. Microadenoma ($\leq$10 mm)
2. Macroadenoma (>10 mm)

Growth Pattern

1. Expansive. Growth of an adenoma results in compression of acini in surrounding pituitary tissue (Fig. 1). Significant growth causes displacement of the posterior lobe, pituitary stalk (see stalk section effect above), or optic chiasm, as well as compressive expansion of the bony sella. It is of note that diabetes insipidus rarely results, despite significant displacement of the pituitary stalk and often marked compression of the posterior lobe by large adenomas.

2. Grossly invasive of dura, bone, nerves, and brain. Invasiveness of pituitary adenomas is predicated on radiographic or gross (opera-

tive) findings. Note: Due to its high frequency of occurrence in both micro- and macroadenomas, the simple demonstration of microscopic dural infiltration is not considered to be clinically significant. Involvement of vessels and nerves is generally limited to adventitial and perineural invasion. The demonstration of brain invasion, a feature of malignancy in adenohypophyseal tumours, is virtually limited to autopsy examination.

3. Metastasising (craniospinal or systemic). Metastasis is the *sine qua non* of malignancy in pituitary tumours. Spread is just as often craniospinal as systemic and frequently includes both modes. The diagnosis of pituitary carcinoma must be morphologically confirmed, preferably with immunohistochemical and/or ultrastructural support.

2   Tumours of the Adrenal Cortex

2.1   Adrenal Cortical Tumours

2.1.1   Benign

2.1.1.1 Adrenal Cortical Adenoma (Figs. 25–29)

A benign neoplasm of adrenal cortical cells.

Adrenal cortical adenoma (ACA) grows in nests (Fig. 25), short cords, or trabeculae (Fig. 26) or uncommonly in a diffuse (solid) growth pattern. In some tumours, there may be an admixture of these patterns. Tumour cells are usually larger than cells of the normal cortical zones but may resemble them with respect to the amount of cytoplasmic lipid (pale-staining or lipid-rich versus compact or lipid-poor), nuclear morphology, and presence or absence of lipofuscin. Cells with pale-staining lipid-rich cytoplasm usually predominate, and occasionally there may be balloon cells with abundant cytoplasmic lipid.

In ACAs associated with primary hyperaldosteronism (Table 7) there may be cells morphologically resembling those of the zona fasciculata and zona glomerulosa as well as cells with compact lipid-poor cytoplasm resembling zona reticularis-type cells. Hybrid cells have been described which are intermediate between glomerulosa and fasciculata-type cells. ACAs associated with virilisation often have a predominance of cells with compact lipid-poor cytoplasm. As a general rule, however, the presence of any particular architectural or cytological feature is not completely reliable in predicting the presence or absence of an endocrine syndrome; and close correlation with clinical and/or endocrinological data is indicated. There may be some very helpful clues in suspecting an associated syndrome such as the atrophy of attached or contralateral adrenal cortex which regularly occurs with Cushing syndrome (Fig. 27). In primary hyperaldosteronism, the presence of hyperplasia of zona glomerulosa (Fig. 28) or in patients treated with the aldosterone antagonist spironolactone, the occurrence of scroll-like eosinophilic inclusions may provide a clue.

Nuclear enlargement with hyperchromasia and pleomorphism can be found in some ACAs (Fig. 29), but it is not a reliable criterion for predicting biologic behaviour. Mitotic figures are rare in ACA, particularly atypical mitoses. Foci of lipomatous or myelolipomatous metaplasia may be present, but are usually a minor component within the tumour. Rarely, one may find intracytoplasmic hyaline globules similar to those of pheochromocytoma (Fig. 26). On occasion, it may be very difficult to distinguish an adrenal cortical neoplasm from a pheochromocytoma. Features common to both and contributing to this include 1) alveolar (or nesting) pattern, 2) compact eosinophilic to amphophilic cytoplasm, 3) nuclear irregularities, 4) intracytoplasmic hyaline globules, and 5) positive immunostaining for synaptophysin, a neuroendocrine marker. Immunostaining for chromogranin A is regularly negative in adrenal cortical neoplasms.

ACAs usually weigh less than 50 g and are less than 5 cm in diameter. Most ACAs are unilateral, solitary, and well circumscribed; and on cross section they are often yellow-orange due to the presence of abundant lipid-rich cells. The colour may vary considerably in part of or throughout the tumour due to lipid depletion, prominent intracellular lipofuscin, or secondary degenerative change such as haemorrhage. Some tumours may be light brown to jet black throughout. A large proportion of adrenal cortical adenomas (ACAs) are nonfunctional or non*hyper*functional without a clinically detectable endocrine syndrome or biochemical evidence of hypercorticalism (Table 7). It may be discovered incidentally in a nononcological setting, or it may enter into a staging workup of a patient with known malignancy elsewhere. ACA can be a cause of primary (endogenous) hypercorticalism, most often primary hyperaldosteronism (Conn syndrome), followed by Cushing syndrome and occasionally virilisation. The clinical syndrome is usually in "pure" form, but on occasion it may be "mixed", e.g., mixed Cushing syndrome and virilisation. The presence of a mixed endocrine syndrome, virilisation, or feminisation in particular may be cause for concern regarding potential malignancy, and correlation with histologic and nonhistological parameters is indicated.

2.1.1.2 Pigmented ("black") adenoma (Fig. 30)

An adrenal cortical adenoma containing such abundant intracytoplasmic lipofuscin that the tumour appears macroscopically dark brown to black.

These are uncommon tumours and have been reported in association with Cushing syndrome, less commonly primary hyperaldosteronism. There appears to be no clinical significance attached to this accumulation of pigment.

2.1.1.3 Oncocytic adrenal cortical adenoma (Fig. 31)

An adrenal cortical adenoma with cells having abundant compact eosinophilic cytoplasm which is finely granular.

These rare tumours may be clinically nonfunctional. Recent immunohistochemical study has reported decreased activity of enzymes involved in steroidogenesis. Ultrastructural study has shown numerous mitochondria and little to no lipid droplets.

2.1.2   Malignant

2.1.2.1 Adrenal cortical carcinoma (Figs. 32–36)

A malignant neoplasm of adrenal cortical cells.

Histologically the same basic architectural patterns can be found in adrenal cortical carcinoma (ACC) as in ACA; the trabecular pattern, however, can be more conspicuous with broad columns of cells separated by elongate vascular channels or gaping sinusoids (Fig. 32). Occasionally, one may find a ribbon-like or gyriform pattern; a diffuse or solid pattern may predominate in some tumours (Fig. 33). Broad fibrous bands may be present particularly in tumours which have coarse nodularity. Most ACCs are composed of cells with compact eosinophilic cytoplasm. Nuclear enlargement with hyperchromasia and pleomorphism can be a conspicuous feature in ACCs (Fig. 34), but by itself is not reliable in classifying the neoplasm as malignant. Rarely, an ACC can have a myxoid pattern (Fig. 35). Mi-

Table 7. Functional classification of tumours of the adrenal cortex

1	Nonfunctional or nonhyperfunctional
2	Endocrine hyperfunction (hypercorticalism)
2.1	Hypercortisolism (Cushing syndrome)
2.2	Hyperaldosteronism (Conn syndrome)
2.3	Virilisation
2.4	Feminisation
2.5	Mixed endocrine syndrome
3	Functional status unknown

totic activity (usually ≥6 per 50 high power fields), atypical mitoses, and vascular invasion in some studies have been shown to be most predictive of malignant behaviour. Markers of cellular proliferation (e.g., Ki 67) may provide useful information. Regional or distant metastases have been noted in a small but significant number of patients at time of presentation. Similar to ACAs, intracytoplasmic hyaline globules can also be found in ACCs (Fig. 34). Lipomatous and myelolipomatous metaplasia can occur but is rare. It is important to note that many ACCs can show strong immunoreactivity for synaptophysin, which may invite confusion with pheochromocytoma (Fig. 36).

Adrenal cortical carcinoma (ACC) is usually a large tumour, over 5 cm in diameter and often weighing well over 100 g, but exceptions do occur. Some very large tumours (e.g., 1000 g or more) fail to metastasise or recur, while, rarely, some very small tumours (e.g., less than 50 g) prove to be malignant. On gross inspection, ACCs may be coarsely nodular on cross-section with zones of haemorrhage and geographic necrosis. There may be evidence of extracapsular extension or invasion of adjacent organs. Adrenal cortical carcinoma can be clinically functional and associated with any of the endocrine syndromes noted for ACAs (Table 7). Adrenal cortical neoplasms associated with feminisation are usually classified as ACC. Primary hyperaldosteronism is very uncommon with ACC, occurring in less than 5% of tumours. In some cases, it may be very difficult using gross, microscopic, and other features to clearly separate benign tumours from malignant adrenal cortical tumours.

2.1.2.2 Adrenal carcinosarcoma

A rare malignant neoplasm of adrenal cortex showing mixed mesenchymal ingredients, such as spindle cell sarcoma, in addition to adrenal cortical carcinoma.

An example of adrenal cortical "blastoma" has also been reported.

2.2   Adrenal Cortical Nodules and Tumour-like Lesions

2.2.1   *Nodular adrenal cortical hyperplasia* (Figs. 37, 38)

One or more nodules of non-neoplastic adrenal cortical cells which may form a macroscopically visible lesion or dominant macronodule simulating a neoplasm.

Nodular adrenal cortical hyperplasia is, in most cases, bilateral and may be symmetric or asymmetric. Micronodules and macronodules have been recognised, but the distinction based upon size is arbitrary. Some have designated macronodules as being ≥1 cm, others equate a macronodule as being any size detectable on computed tomographic (CT) scan and others as any nodules detectable on gross inspection of the gland. The nodular adrenal gland can present a confusing clinical and pathologic picture, particularly when there is a dominant macronodule or, occasionally, when bilateral macronodules are present. The patient is characteristically eucortical without clinical or endocrinological evidence of excess corticosteroid secretion. Some patients with excess ACTH stimulation may develop one or more hyperplastic adrenal cortical nodules (e.g., Cushing syndrome and congenital adrenal hyperplasia). The morphological distinction between a dominant macronodule and nonfunctioning ACA can be difficult and even arbitrary. The range in histology of nodular hyperplasia can mimic that seen in adrenal cortical neoplasms (Figs. 37, 38). Nodular hyperplasia may be accompanied by diffuse hyperplasia.

2.2.2   *Heterotopic and accessory adrenal cortical nodules*
(Figs. 39, 40)

Nonneoplastic adrenal cortical tissue located in an extra-adrenal site

Heterotopic adrenal cortical nodules can be found anywhere along the path of gonadal descent in both sexes. The nodule may occur in periadrenal connective tissue beneath the capsule of the kidney (usually upper pole), in the celiac axis, near the fallopian tube and ovary (Fig. 39), along the vas deferens and hilum of the testis, but has been reported in anatomic sites defying simple embryological explanation (e.g., lung and placenta). The nodule is usually solitary and, in sites removed from the adrenal glands and celiac axis, is usually composed of cortical cells without a medullary component. The nodules are usually small (<5 mm), sharply circumscribed or encapsulated, and have cytoarchitecture which may or may not resemble zonation seen in the eutopic adrenal. Rarely, accessory cortical tissue has been reported in parenchyma of ovary and testis. Heterotopic and accessory adrenal cortical tissue may become enlarged and hyperplastic with excess ACTH stimulation (e.g., congenital adrenal hyperplasia or adrenogenital syndrome). Rarely, a true adrenal cortical neoplasm can arise in heterotopic or accessory adrenal cortical tissue.

Small nodules of accessory adrenal cortical tissue can be seen as extrusions on the surface of the adrenal glands which may or may not be encapsulated, and in the plane of section may or may not show a connection with underlying cortex. The configuration is sometimes likened to a mushroom or door handle (Fig. 40). Cortical extrusions may also become hyperplastic.

2.2.3 Primary pigmented nodular adrenocortical disease (Figs. 41, 42)

A rare pituitary or ACTH-independent form of Cushing syndrome where adrenal glands may be small, normal in size, or enlarged and usually contain multiple pigmented cortical nodules.

Primary pigmented nodular adrenocortical disease (PPNAD) usually affects young individuals. The adrenal glands are small, normal in size, or slightly enlarged and have bilateral, small, brown to black nodules studding the cortex. Occasionally, there may be one or more macronodules. Some nodules may be pale yellow to tan.

The aetiology of PPNAD is uncertain, but it is a rare autonomous cause of Cushing syndrome which is non-neoplastic. Immunohistochemical studies have demonstrated increased immunoreactivity for enzymes involved in steroidogenesis, helping to explain why glands small, normal, or slightly increased in size can cause hypercortisolism.

2.2.4   Macronodular hyperplasia
with marked adrenal enlargement (Figs. 43, 44)

A rare pituitary or ACTH-independent form of Cushing syndrome where both adrenal glands are typically enlarged, due to nodular hyperplasia.

Macronodular hyperplasia with marked adrenal enlargement (MHMAE) is another rare cause of Cushing syndrome in which sensitive imaging and dynamic endocrinological testing indicate a primary adrenal cause of hypercortisolism. Both adrenal glands are enlarged (combined weight usually over 80 g) and grossly may simulate a neoplasm.

Individual macronodules have histomorphology which overlaps that seen in nodular hyperplasia. Immunohistochemical studies have shown weak immunoreactivity for enzymes involved in steroidogenesis, suggesting that marked hyperplasia must exist before hypercortisolism becomes manifest. The aetiology of MHMAE is uncertain. Some suggest that it may be related to long-standing Cushing syndrome (pituitary or ACTH-dependent hypercortisolism) which, over time, becomes adrenal-dependent or autonomous.

2.2.5   Adrenal cytomegaly (Fig. 45)

Nuclear enlargement and hyperchromasia of foetal (provisional) cortical cells which can be focal or diffuse.

Adrenal cytomegaly is a characteristic feature of the Beckwith-Wiedemann syndrome. Mitotic figures are characteristically absent. The aetiology is unclear but does not appear related to neoplasia.

2.3   Other Adrenal Neoplasms and Tumour-like Lesions

2.3.1   Benign

2.3.1.1 Myelolipoma (Fig. 46)

A tumefactive lesion of the adrenal composed of mature adipose tissue and haematopoietic elements in various proportion.

Myelolipoma presents as a unilateral mass (rarely bilateral) which varies in size and colour, ranging from yellow to red-brown, depending upon the proportion and admixture of fat and haematopoietic tissue. Myelolipomas can occur in a variety of extra-adrenal sites. The fatty component is mature adipose tissue, and there is often trilinear composition of haematopoietic cells, including megakaryocytes. Lipomatous and myelolipomatous metaplasia can be found in a variety of adrenal cortical disorders, both hyperplastic and neoplastic.

2.3.1.2 Adrenal cyst

A benign cystic lesion of adrenal gland which can cause tumefactive enlargement.

Adrenal cysts have been divided into vascular, epithelial, and parasitic types. Adrenal pseudocyst, the most common encountered clinically, has no apparent lining, although with further study, including immunohistochemistry, some of these have been shown to be vascular or epithelial cysts. Rarely, an adrenal neoplasm such as cystic pheochromocytoma can mimic an adrenal cyst.

2.3.1.3 Primary mesenchymal tumours

Hemangioma, leiomyoma, lipoma, and solitary fibrous tumours occur.

2.3.1.4 Other

Adenomatoid tumour (Fig. 47) is a very unusual primary neoplasm of the adrenal gland which, by immunohistochemical and ultrastructural study, has been shown to be a mesothelioma. The tumour has a microcystic or pseudoglandular pattern which insinuates between cords and nests of cortical cells.

Sex cord-stromal tumours have rarely been documented. Very unusual adrenal neoplasms containing Leydig (or hilus) cells with identifiable crystalloids of Reincke have been described and may be associated with masculinisation. A case of adrenal *granulosa cell tumour* has been reported. Also noted is a small incidental lesion, *ovarian thecal metaplasia*, which occurs in females (but not exclusively) and resembles theca cells of the ovary. It has no known association with neoplasia. *Tumefactive spindle nodules* have also been reported in the adrenals.

Other tumour-like lesions include adrenal haemorrhage with haematoma formation and some infectious diseases that cause tumefactive enlargement of the adrenal glands (e.g., tuberculosis and histoplasmosis).

2.3.2   Malignant

2.3.2.1 Sarcomas

Angiosarcoma (Fig. 48), leiomyosarcoma, and malignant peripheral nerve sheath tumour have been described as being primary in the adrenal.

2.3.2.2 Other

Rare examples of *malignant lymphoma* have been reported primary in the adrenal gland. *Malignant melanoma* is also a rare primary adrenal tumour which may contain conspicuous melanin pigment or be amelanotic. Care must be taken to distinguish this tumour from a pigmented or *melanotic paraganglioma*.

2.4   Secondary Tumours

The adrenal glands have been reported to be the fourth most common site of metastases, following lung, liver, and bone. If small, the metastasis may be restricted to the cortex or medulla. When large, the metastatic tumour may destroy much of the gland. Bilateral metastatic tumour can result in adrenal cortical insufficiency (Addison disease). Occasionally, metastatic carcinoma can grossly and microscopically mimic an ACC. Common primary sites of metastatic carcinoma are lung and breast. The adrenal glands can also be secondarily involved by sarcomas, but this is very unusual.

2.5   Unclassified Tumours

3   Tumours of Adrenal and Extra-adrenal Paraganglia

Sympathoadrenal paraganglia and parasympathetic paraganglia of the head and neck region are part of a diffuse neuroendocrine system which plays different physiological roles in homeostasis. The sympathoadrenal neuroendocrine system has a roughly symmetric distribution along the paravertebral axis, extending from high in the neck near the superior cervical ganglion down into the abdomen and true pelvis, and may have small paraganglia associated with organs such as urinary bladder and prostate gland. The largest, most compact collection of paraganglia in this system is the adrenal medulla on either side. This neuroendocrine system is involved in making rapid adaptations to changes in the environment, and the effects are dissipated rather quickly. Physiologic effects are mediated by the neurotransmitter norepinephrine (NE), released from postganglionic sympathetic nerve endings, and by the hormone epinephrine (E), which is synthesised and released by the adrenal medullae, as well as a lesser amount of NE (a hormone as well as a neurotransmitter).

Paraganglia of the head and neck region and some in the middle mediastinum have a closer alignment with the parasympathetic nervous system and some have spatial relationship with branchial arch mesodermal derivatives (i.e., carotid body paraganglia). Some paraganglia within this neuroendocrine system have been shown experimentally to have a chemoreceptor function by sensing alterations in paO_2, $paCO_2$, and pH with reflex alterations in breathing and cardiovascular function. A significant increase in incidence of carotid body paraganglioma ("chemodectoma" – chemeia: "infusion"–; deschesthai: "to receive" –; and oma: "tumour") has been reported in humans dwelling at high altitude (e.g., the Peruvian Andes). The largest, most compact collections of paraganglia in the head and neck region are the carotid bodies, with the average normal combined weight in adults being a little over 12 mg. Paraganglia are also distributed near the skull base (jugular and vagal paraganglia), the middle ear (tympanic paraganglia), larynx, and base of heart in relation to great vessels. Carotid body chief cells have been shown to contain dopamine with lesser amounts of NE and only trace quantities of E.

A neural crest origin has been firmly established for carotid body chief cells and chromaffin cells of the adrenal medulla, and identical embryological derivation is presumed for other endocrine cells of the paraganglionic system. Tumours of the sympathoadrenal neuroendocrine system are often functionally active (and may be chromaffin-positive), with secretion of catecholamines in various combinations, while tumours of head and neck paraganglia are characteristically endocrinologically silent (typically chromaffin-negative), although rare exceptions exist. Some tumours arising from aorticopulmonary paraganglia can cause excess catecholamine secretion. Cytoplasmic argyrophilia may be useful in diagnosis using techniques such as the Grimelius stain. Paraganglionic chief cells (characteristically nonchromaffin), as well as their neoplastic counterparts, are typically immunoreactive for neuroendocrine markers such as chromogranin A, synaptophysin, and neuron-specific enolase. Immunostaining for neuroendocrine markers such as chromogranin can be particularly helpful in diagnosis of these tumours. Electron microscopy may also provide valuable diagnostic information through detection of dense-core neurosecretory granules. Another cell type which occurs in normal paraganglia as well as tumours derived from them is the sustentacular cell, which characteristically shows immunoreactivity for S-100 protein and appears as a plump spindle or dendritic cell at the edge of cords and nests of endocrine cells.

3.1   Paragangliomas

3.1.1   Sympathoadrenal paragangliomas

3.1.1.1 Pheochromocytoma (adrenal medullary paraganglioma) (Figs. 49–55)

A paraganglioma arising from chromaffin cells of adrenal medulla. (The term pheochromocytoma has also been applied to extra-adrenal paragangliomas of the sympathoadrenal neuroendocrine system.)
      Pheochromocytoma is usually solitary, unilateral, and unicentric. Pheochromocytomas in a familial setting such as multiple endocrine neoplasia (MEN) syndromes type 2a and 2b are frequently bilateral and may be multicentric or multinodular. The precursor to development of pheochromocytoma(s) in this familial setting is adrenal medullary hyperplasia which may be diffuse and/or nodular. Although circumscribed and appearing encapsulated, some tumours have a fibrous pseudocapsule from compression of adjacent connective tissue or acquire a capsule from expansion of the adrenal gland. The cut surface of pheochromocytomas varies from grey, tan to red-brown, and some may be markedly haemorrhagic. Occasionally, central areas of degeneration are present, and some of the larger tumours may be-

come cystic. Immersion in appropriate dichromate containing fixative may elicit a characteristic chromaffin reaction, but this is not essential for diagnosis. Pheochromocytomas have architectural patterns which can be broadly classified as alveolar (nesting), anastomosing cell cord (or trabecular) (Figs. 49, 50), and diffuse (or solid). Tumour cells are polygonal or fusiform, and some tumours have a spindle cell pattern which is usually focal (Fig. 51). There may be a moderate to marked degree of nuclear pleomorphism, and nuclear pseudoinclusions can be found in some tumours (Fig. 52), a reflection of infolding or irregularity of the nuclear membrane with inward extension of cell cytoplasm. Cells have amphophilic to lightly eosinophilic, finely granular cytoplasm. In some tumours, the cytoplasm is lilac or lavender with a myriad of pinpoint granules (Fig. 53), many of which represent neurosecretory type granules. Intracytoplasmic hyaline globules which are PAS-positive can be found in many pheochromocytomas (Fig. 54), but they may be difficult to find on casual inspection. Identical hyaline globules can be seen in the normal adrenal medulla in many cases. At times, the histomorphology of pheochromocytoma strongly resembles that of the normal adrenal medulla. At the interface with adjacent cortex, the tumour may appear unencapsulated with some intermingling of cortical cells, a feature which can also be seen in the normal adrenal gland. An increased incidence of periadrenal brown fat has been reported.

There are no single or combined morphologic findings which predict malignant behaviour, aside from documentation of metastases to anatomic sites where paraganglia do not normally reside. The presence of a combination of extensive necrosis, readily identifiable mi-

Table 8. Functional classification of tumours of adrenal and extra-adrenal paraganglia

1	Functional disturbance
1.1	Hypofunction[a]
1.2	Hyperfunction
1.2.1	Hypertension
1.2.2	Diarrhoea
1.2.3	Cushing syndrome
1.2.4	Others, such as acromegaly
2	No functional disturbance
3	Functional state undetermined

[a] Hypothetical at present, since there is no known adrenoprival syndrome due to deficiency of adrenal medulla or extra-adrenal paraganglia.

totic figures, or vascular invasion are suggestive of more aggressive behaviour but are not *per se* diagnostic of malignancy. These tumours characteristically elicit signs and/or symptoms of excess catecholamine secretion and on rare occasions have caused Cushing syndrome, due to ectopic secretion of adrenocorticotropic hormone (ACTH) or a watery diarrhoea syndrome due to vasoactive intestinal peptide (VIP) secretion (Table 8).

3.1.1.2 Extra-adrenal paraganglioma

A paraganglioma arising from extra-adrenal paraganglia of the sympathoadrenal neuroendocrine system.

These tumours are mostly intra-abdominal and may arise from remnants of the organs of Zuckerkandl, which are paraganglia distributed on either side of the aorta from the level of the superior mesenteric artery down to the aortic bifurcation. Paragangliomas may also arise in the urinary bladder and other sites in the abdomen, as well as in the filum terminale. Paragangliomas parallel the distribution of the paravertebral sympathetic chain and occasionally occur in the thorax and rarely the neck. These paragangliomas may be functionally active with excess secretion of catecholamines (usually NE or dopamine). Their histologic appearance mirrors that of pheochromocytomas. Designation by anatomical site of origin is the preferred mode of classification. Rarely, extra-adrenal paragangliomas have been reported to be pigmented or melanotic (Fig. 55).

3.1.1.3 Composite pheochromocytoma
or extra-adrenal paraganglioma

A tumour that combines features of typical paraganglioma (adrenal or extra-adrenal) with a component resembling neuroblastoma or ganglioneuroblastoma (Figs. 56–58) or have a well-developed growth pattern of ganglioneuroma (Fig. 59); rarely there may be a malignant peripheral nerve sheath tumour.

Composite pheochromocytomas are rare tumours which combine both neural and endocrine features. Some pheochromocytomas may have cells with neuronal or ganglionic features and, when well-developed and combined with neuritic processes and abundance of a pale fibrillar material resembling neuropil, the tumour resembles a pattern seen in neuroblastoma and ganglioneuroblastoma. The resemblance to a less mature neuroblastic tumour does not necessarily equate with malignant behaviour, and the biology of these tumours can be as difficult to predict as the usual paraganglioma.

3.1.2   Paragangliomas of the head and neck region

Paragangliomas arising from paraganglia often having close alignment or relation with the parasympathetic nervous system.

The most common paragangliomas in the head and neck are carotid body, jugulotympanic, vagal, and laryngeal paragangliomas, although histologically identical tumours can occur at the base of the heart in relation to the great vessels (aorticopulmonary paragangliomas) and in other sites (e.g., orbit). On purely histologic grounds, these tumours may be very difficult to distinguish one from the other without knowledge of anatomical site of origin, and comments about morphology will concentrate briefly on the prototypical tumour in this group, carotid body paraganglioma (CBP or "chemodectoma").

3.1.2.1 Carotid body paraganglioma (CBP) (Figs. 60–62)

A paraganglioma arising from carotid body paraganglia located in or near the bifurcation of the common carotid artery.

These tumours, along with other paragangliomas of the head and neck region, tend to have a well-developed nesting (or alveolar) pattern often referred to as "zellballen" (Fig. 60). This organoid nesting pattern can be greatly accentuated by staining for reticulum (Fig. 61) or neuroendocrine markers such as chromogranin A (Fig. 62). CBP and other head and neck paragangliomas only vaguely mirror the histomorphology of the corresponding non-neoplastic paraganglion. The basic neoplastic element is the chief cell, which is often ovoid or polygonal and larger than the non-neoplastic chief cell. Cell borders may be indistinct. Cytoplasm is lightly eosinophilic and often finely granular. Occasionally, a CBP may contain cells with abundant eosinophilic granular cytoplasm. Nuclear hyperchromasia and pleomorphism may be seen but are not useful in predicting prognosis. Occasionally, some "zellballen" may be enlarged with central degeneration or necrosis.

Stromal alterations may occur, such as sclerosis (more common in vagal and jugulotympanic paragangliomas), sinusoidal telangiectasis, and evidence of recent and old haemorrhage. There is also a population of sustentacular cells best appreciated by immunostain for S-100 protein (Fig. 63); these cells regularly escape detection in routinely stained sections, and can also be present in sites of local spread or distant metastases. CBP and other paragangliomas of the head and neck are only rarely functional with excess catecholamine secretion. There are no reliable morphologic criteria which can predict biological behaviour.

CBP is usually unilateral and solitary in a sporadic setting but, with familial occurrence, may be bilateral and/or associated with other paragangliomas in the head and neck region. The tumours are usually well-circumscribed and, when small, form a discrete mass in the widened carotid bifurcation; larger tumours can surround or envelop the bifurcation and carotid vessels. CBP may appear encapsulated, but this is best regarded as a fibrous pseudocapsule.

3.1.2.2 Jugulotympanic paraganglioma (Fig. 63)

A paraganglioma arising from dispersed paraganglia in the skull base and middle ear.

This tumour can sometimes be subdivided into jugular paraganglioma arising from dispersed paraganglia at the skull base, often in association with the adventitia of the jugular bulb, and tympanic paraganglioma, a tumour of the middle ear, particularly the promontory. When the tumour is large or obscures normal anatomical landmarks, the term "jugulotympanic" may be preferred. The tumour may spread along bony fissures, crevices, and foramina and can invade bone.

3.1.2.3 Vagal paraganglioma

A paraganglioma arising from dispersed paraganglia located in the rostral vagus nerve, often close to the ganglion nodosum.

3.1.2.4 Laryngeal paraganglioma

A paraganglioma arising from dispersed paraganglia associated with the larynx.

3.1.2.5 Aorticopulmonary paraganglioma

A paraganglioma arising from dispersed paraganglia located at the base of the heart and associated with great vessels.

These tumours arise from paraganglia located at the base of the heart and in relation to great vessels. They may be divided into cardiac and extracardiac paragangliomas, depending upon precise location. A significant proportion of these tumours may be functionally active with excess catecholamine release, suggesting a closer alignment of some of these tumours with the sympathetic nervous system.

3.1.2.6 Other paragangliomas

These include paragangliomas of the orbit, pterygoid fossa, etc.

3.1.3   Paraganglioma, not further classified

3.2   Neural and Neuroblastic Tumours

3.2.1   Benign

These tumours are histologically identical to tumours arising in other extra-adrenal sites. Adrenal neurofibroma and neurilemoma have been reported, but ganglioneuroma, ganglioneuroblastoma, and neuroblastoma are the most important ones to consider.

3.2.1.1 Ganglioneuroma (Figs. 64–66)

A benign tumour composed of ganglion cells in various proportions, which may be immature or dysmorphic (e.g., multinucleation and nuclear pyknosis), and Schwann cells.

Ganglion cells vary greatly in number and distribution (Fig. 64). Nuclei are usually eccentric and vesicular with a prominent nucleolus. Cytoplasm is usually well-defined, abundant, eosinophilic, and may show Nissl substance at the periphery. Granular pigment consistent with neuromelanin may be seen in some ganglion cells (Fig. 65). Occasionally, there are satellite cells adjacent to ganglion cells. The spindle cell schwannian matrix may be loose and fascicular. Clusters of lymphocytes may be present and should not be misinterpreted as neuroblasts (Fig. 66).

3.2.2   Malignant

3.2.2.1/3.2.2.2   Neuroblastoma and ganglioneuroblastoma (Figs. 67–70)

Tumours arising from primitive cells of neural crest origin which may be undifferentiated or show varying degrees of maturation into ganglion cells and/or a spindle cell schwannian matrix.

These tumours show a veritable continuum in differentiation, with the most immature being primitive neuroblastoma (NB) without any evidence of ganglion cell differentiation, while the most mature tumours show such a high level of differentiation that they may be mistakenly classified as ganglioneuroma. Differentiation is defined by the acquisition of ganglion cell cytomorphology with nuclear enlargement, increased cytoplasmic eosinophilia, and well-defined cell borders. Most current views do not recognise Homer Wright rosettes or a matted fibrillary matrix as evidence of differentiation for prognostic grouping.

Histologically, NB can be composed of sheets of primitive cells (Fig. 67) lacking any evidence of ganglion cell differentiation and have scant to undetectable fibrillary matrix (the latter represents aggregated or intertwined neuritic processes). A vague, lobular growth pattern is characteristic with delicate fibrovascular septa. There may be Homer Wright rosettes with a rounded pale fibrillar centre composed of a tangled skein of neuritic cell processes (Fig. 68). A rare tumour may have palisaded rosettes. Some tumours contain abundant matted fibrillary matrix resembling neuropil (Fig. 69). In recent grading classifications, undifferentiated NB is defined as a tumour containing fewer than 5% ganglion cells, while differentiating NB contains more (Fig. 70). Nuclei of neuroblasts are usually round to ovoid with dispersed nuclear chromatin likened to salt and pepper. Occasionally, nuclear pleomorphism is present, but it does not appear to have an adverse effect on prognosis. Ultrastructural demonstration of neurosecretory granules, microtubules, and neurofilaments may be useful in diagnosis.

Grossly, NB often has a soft encephaloid consistency with bulging friable lobules showing areas of haemorrhage and necrosis. Dystrophic calcification, which often develops in the wake of tumour necrosis, can sometimes be appreciated as punctate areas of opacity and may be a prominent feature in some tumours. This finding has been cited as a favourable morphologic finding in NB and ganglioneuroblastoma (GNB) in a recent grading system. As the tumour differentiates, it may acquire a rich complement of a spindle cell schwannian matrix. Using the Shimada age-linked classification[1], such tumours are classified as stroma-rich and subdivided into three groups: well-differentiated, intermixed, and nodular. Stroma-poor tumours are also recognised. NB and GNB arise in sites paralleling the distribution of the sympathetic nervous system; most tumours are intra-abdominal and usually located in the adrenal gland, but can arise in the posterior thorax or neck.

The Shimada age-linked classification of NB and GNB identified prognostically favourable and unfavourable subgroups. The stroma-rich tumours have a prominent component of spindle cell schwannian matrix. Three subtypes are recognised – well-differentiated, intermixed and nodular. There is a stroma-poor category which is stratified using age at diagnosis, proportion of differentiating cells, and mitosis-karyorrhexis index (MKI). Favourable subgroups include patients with stroma-rich, well-differentiated, and intermixed tumours, and the stroma-poor tumours which have low MKI, more than 5% differentiating elements, and young age at diagnosis. The unfavourable subgroups include patients with nodular stroma-rich tumours (also referred to as composite ganglioneuroblastoma) and stroma-poor tumours which have a high MKI, less than 5% differentiating elements, and older age at diagnosis. More recent classification or modified grading schemes have utilised a combination of age at diagnosis, proportion of differentiating elements, and presence or absence of calcification to stratify prognostic subgroups[2]. NB and GNB have been reported to undergo spontaneous or treatment-induced maturation or regression; occasionally, the maturation endpoint is completely mature ganglioneuroma. A special category of patients with neuroblastoma is recognised (Stage IV patients) where prognosis is remarkably favourable, despite an impressive tumour

---

[1] Shimada H, Chatten J, Newton WA Jr et al. (1984) Histopathologic factors in neuroblastic tumours: definition of subtypes of ganglioneuroblastoma and an age-linked classification of neuroblastomas. J Natl Cancer Inst 73:405–416

[2] Joshi VV, Cantor AB, Altshuler G et al.(1992) Age-linked prognostic categorisation based on a new histologic grading system of neuroblastomas: a clinicopathologic study of 211 cases from the Pediatric Oncology Group. Cancer 69: 2197–2211

burden involving liver, skin, and bone marrow; these children are usually under the age of one year at diagnosis. Some tumours may secrete substances, such as catecholamines, which may cause hypertension or vasoactive intestinal peptide which has been associated with watery diarrhoea.

3.2.2.3 Primitive neuroectodermal tumour

This primitive tumour with neural phenotype occurs more commonly in soft tissue and bone. Cytogenetic analysis may aid in diagnosis.

3.2.2.4 Malignant peripheral nerve sheath tumour (malignant schwannoma)

3.2.2.5 Primitive neural neoplasm, not otherwise classified

3.3   Unclassified Tumours

3.4   Tumour-like Lesions

3.4.1   Adrenal medullary hyperplasia

Rarely, this may be the cause of systemic hypertension in a sporadic setting and forms the precursor lesion of pheochromocytomas in MEN syndromes types 2a and 2b. It may be diffuse and/or nodular and difficult to distinguish from an early pheochromocytoma. Identification of early medullary hyperplasia may be very difficult and require methodical use of morphometric analysis of well-oriented transverse sections of adrenal gland(s), concentrating on the head and body where chromaffin tissue is most abundant. Lesions over 1 cm in diameter have been arbitrarily designated pheochromocytoma.

3.4.2   Hyperplasia of extra-adrenal paraganglia

Hyperplasia has been best characterised for carotid body paraganglia in high altitude dwellers and patients at or near sea level with chronic hypoxemia due to chronic obstructive pulmonary disease, cyanotic congenital heart disease, and cystic fibrosis. Tumefactive enlargement has been reported in patients dwelling at high altitude.

3.4.3   Neuroblastic nodules (Fig. 71)

Neuroblastic nodules are a normal part of embryogenesis and development of the foetal adrenal gland, and may linger until birth or early infancy. They enter into the differential diagnosis of in situ neuroblastoma.

4   Tumours of the Parathyroid Glands

4.1   Adenoma

A benign encapsulated neoplasm composed of chief cells, oncocytes, transitional oncocytes, or admixtures of these cell types.

Most parathyroid adenomas are functional (Table 9) and are responsible for 85% of cases of primary hyperparathyroidism in most large case series. Approximately 90% of adenomas involve the upper or lower glands of the neck, while the remainder occur in a variety of other sites including the mediastinum, retro-oesophageal soft tissue, thyroid, and thymus. Rarely, adenomas may arise from ectopic or supernumerary parathyroid tissue within the pericardium, the vagus nerve, or soft tissues adjacent to the angle of the jaw. The distinction of parathyroid adenoma from hyperplasia requires examination of at least one additional gland, which should be normal in cases of adenoma. However, rare examples of double adenomas have been reported.

4.1.1   Chief cell adenoma (Figs. 72–80)

A benign encapsulated neoplasm composed predominantly or exclusively of chief cells.

Table 9. Functional classification of tumours and tumour-like lesions of the parathyroid glands

1	Nonfunctional
2	Hyperfunctional
2.1	Hyperparathyroidism
3	Hypofunctional
3.1	Hypoparathyroidism
4	Functional status unknown

A rim of normal parathyroid tissue is present in 50%–60% of cases of parathyroid adenoma. The probability of finding a normal rim of parathyroid, however, decreases with increasing size of the tumour (Figs. 72, 73). The neoplastic chief cells may be arranged in cords, nests, or diffuse sheets (Figs. 73-75). A follicular (glandular) pattern may be present focally or may be the predominant pattern throughout the tumour (Fig. 76, 77). The follicular lumens may contain an eosinophilic colloid-like material which often stains positively with Congo red. Rare examples of papillary chief cell adenomas may also occur. In cases with a sheet-like pattern of growth, the tumour cells often have a palisaded arrangement around blood vessels. The distinction between chief cell adenoma and hyperplasia requires the examination of at least one additional gland which should be normal in cases of adenoma and hypercellular in cases of hyperplasia.

Neoplastic chief cells are often larger than the chief cells present in the adjacent normal parathyroid tissue. The cytoplasm is faintly eosinophilic but may appear clear (Figs. 74, 75). In some instances, oncocytes may be admixed with the chief cells (Fig. 78). The nuclei are generally round with dense chromatin and occasional small nucleoli. Mitotic figures may be present but are generally sparse. Chief cells with enlarged hyperchromatic nuclei may be dispersed throughout the tumour or present in small foci (Fig. 79). Adenoma cells generally contain little or no intracytoplasmic neutral lipid. If present, lipid deposits tend to be finely dispersed. Neutral lipid deposits tend to be larger in normal chief cells adjacent to the adenoma or in a second parathyroid gland (Fig. 73).

Nodular aggregates of relatively pure populations of chief cells with more or less cytoplasm than the remaining chief cells comprising the bulk of the adenoma may be present. The cells within the nodules have a higher proliferative fraction than the adjacent chief cells.

Foci of cystic degeneration are common, particularly in larger tumours. Degenerative changes are often accompanied by fibrosis and haemosiderin deposition. Entrapment of neoplastic chief cells may occur within the capsules of adenomas with cystic degeneration (Fig. 80). Rarely, chief cell adenomas may undergo spontaneous infarction.

4.1.2   Oncocytic adenoma (Fig. 81)

A benign encapsulated neoplasm composed exclusively or predominantly (more than 90%) of mitochondrion-rich oncocytes.

Individual cells have abundant granular eosinophilic cytoplasm and centrally placed, round to ovoid nuclei with coarsely clumped chromatin and prominent nucleoli. There may be considerable variation in nuclear size, multinucleation, and occasional bizarre hyperchromatic nuclear forms. The oncocytes are typically arranged in cords, nests, broad sheets, or glandular patterns (Fig. 81). The distinction of oncocytic adenoma from hyperplasia requires the examination of at least one additional gland, which should be normal in cases of oncocytic adenoma.

4.1.3   Clear cell adenoma (Fig. 82)

A benign encapsulated neoplasm composed of large polyhedral cells with distinct plasma membranes and extensively vacuolated (water-clear) cytoplasm.

The cells are arranged in short cords and nests with the formation of occasional follicular structures (Fig. 82). The nuclei are round to ovoid and moderately hyperchromatic, with an eccentrically placed nucleolus. The distinction of water-clear cell adenoma from water-clear cell hyperplasia requires the examination of at least one additional gland which should be normal in cases of water-clear cell adenoma.

4.1.4   Lipoadenoma (Fig. 83)

A hamartoma-like benign neoplasm containing both chief cells and prominent stromal elements.

Lipoadenomas are rare and usually associated with hyperparathyroidism, although nonfunctional lipoadenomas have also been described. The parenchymal elements include chief cells and small numbers of oncocytes in a thin, branching, cord-like arrangement (Fig. 83). The cords of chief cells often have a lobular configuration. The stromal compartment includes mature adipose tissue with areas of myxoid change and fibrosis. Prominent collections of lymphocytes are present in some cases.

4.2   Atypical Adenoma (Fig. 84)

A noninvasive parathyroid neoplasm composed of chief cells with variable numbers of oncocytes and transitional oncocytes, with some of the features of parathyroid carcinoma but lacking unequivocal capsular, vascular, or perineural space invasion.

The term "atypical parathyroid adenoma" refers to a neoplasm which has some of the features present in a parathyroid carcinoma but lacks evidence of invasive growth. These features include adherence of tumour to adjacent structures, mitotic activity, fibrosis, trabecular growth pattern, and the presence of tumour cells within the capsule (Fig. 84). In contrast to parathyroid carcinomas, atypical adenomas lack unequivocal capsular, vascular, or perineural space invasion. Atypical adenomas are considered tumours of uncertain malignant potential.

4.3   Carcinoma (Figs. 85–89)

An invasive neoplasm composed of chief cells with variable numbers of oncocytes and transitional oncocytes. Occasional parathyroid carcinomas may be composed exclusively of oncocytes.

Most cases of parathyroid carcinoma are associated with hyperparathyroidism, but occasional cases are nonfunctional (Table 9). The microscopic diagnosis of parathyroid carcinoma is often difficult. Some cases differ minimally from chief cell adenomas, while others are obviously anaplastic (Figs. 85–88). The neoplastic cells may be arranged in cords, nests, diffuse sheets, or trabecular patterns. Principal diagnostic features include thick fibrous bands, mitotic activity, capsular invasion, and vascular invasion. Fibrous bands and mitotic activity, however, are found in substantial numbers of chief cell adenomas. The presence of groups of neoplastic cells entrapped within the capsule is insufficient to warrant a diagnosis of malignancy, since this phenomenon may occur in chief cell adenomas, particularly those with degenerative changes. Invasion of tumour through the capsule with extension into the adjacent soft tissues or thyroid gland, vascular invasion, and perineural space invasion are the most reliable criteria for the diagnosis of malignancy (Fig. 89). The most common sites of metastasis include cervical lymph nodes, lung, and liver.

Analysis of cases lacking invasion and comparison with cases with invasion indicate that fibrosis, necrosis, nuclear atypia with macronucleoli, and mitotic activity are more common in the carcinoma group and correlate positively with aberrant DNA patterns. The presence of macronucleoli, more than five mitoses per 50 high power fields and necrosis are associated with aggressive behaviour. Although mitotic activity is a prognostic factor, it has limited diagnostic significance, since the frequency of mitoses in approximately 50% of the cases of carcinoma does not exceed that found in benign tumours.

Several reports indicate that assessment of proliferative activity by immunohistochemical procedures may predict the behaviour of the tumours. In particular, Ki-67 antigen expressed in more than 6% of the cells is suggestive of carcinoma.

4.4   Tumour-like Lesions

4.4.1   *Primary chief cell hyperplasia* (Figs. 90–92)

An absolute increase in parathyroid parenchymal mass resulting from a proliferation of chief cells, oncocytes, and transitional oncocytes in multiple parathyroid glands in the absence of a recognised stimulus for parathyroid hormone hypersecretion (Table 9).

Symmetric enlargement of all glands occurs in approximately 50% of patients, while the remainder have asymmetric enlargement. The predominant cell in this form of hyperplasia is the chief cell, although variable numbers of oncocytes, transitional oncocytes, and clear cells may be evident. Cellular proliferation may occur either in a nodular or diffuse pattern. The nodular pattern is more common and may be particularly evident in the early phases of the disease. Although hyperplasia is the preferred nomenclature for this disease, molecular studies have established that some of the nodules represent clonal proliferations.

Hyperplastic chief cells may be arranged in cords or nests, sheets, or follicular structures (Fig. 90). Nodules are composed of relatively pure populations of chief cells, oncocytes, transitional oncocytes, or clear cells. The nodules are sharply demarcated from the adjacent diffusely hyperplastic chief cells and are occasionally encapsulated (Figs. 91, 92). Cell proliferation is usually greater in the nodular areas than in the diffusely hyperplastic areas. Hyperplastic chief cells may exhibit slight variation in nuclear size, but pronounced degrees of nuclear pleomorphism are uncommon.

Hyperplastic chief cells typically contain small amounts of intracellular neutral lipid demonstrable with oil red O; however, some hyperplastic glands may contain abundant intracellular fat, at least focally.

Stromal fat cells in cases of primary chief cell hyperplasia are usually markedly reduced; however, because of regional variations in the amount of stromal fat, small biopsies may not be representative and may give spuriously high ratios of stromal fat to parenchymal cells. In some cases, hyperplastic glands contain abundant stromal fat, a change which has been termed "lipohyperplasia".

Chief cell hyperplasia, particularly of the nodular type, may exhibit portions of compressed, mildly hyperplastic parathyroid parenchyma at the gland peripheries, referred to as "pseudorims". Such areas are often impossible to distinguish from a compressed rim of parathyroid tissue adjacent to an adenoma. Although the "pseudorims" should have a relatively small amount of intracellular lipid, some cases contain abundant lipid within the hyperplastic chief cells.

Primary chief cell hyperplasia must be distinguished from parathyroid adenoma, and knowledge of the gross findings is essential for this distinction. In cases of hyperplasia, enlargement of at least two glands is evident, while cases of adenoma typically involve a single gland.

Chronic parathyroiditis is found rarely in association with primary chief cell hyperplasia. Although the origin of the lymphocytic infiltration is unknown, it has been suggested to have an autoimmune origin. Cystic changes in primary chief cell hyperplasia are uncommon and, when they occur, typically involve markedly enlarged glands. Approximately 25% of patients have one of the multiple endocrine neoplasia syndromes or isolated familial hyperparathyroidism, while the remainder have apparent sporadic disease. An unusual familial variant of primary cystic chief cell hyperplasia has also been reported.

4.4.2 Primary (water) clear cell hyperplasia (Fig. 93)

A rare disorder characterised by an absolute increase in parathyroid parenchymal mass resulting from a proliferation of water-clear ("wasserhelle") cells in multiple parathyroid glands in the absence of a known stimulus for parathyroid hormone hypersecretion (Table 9).

All glands are usually enlarged with a greater degree of involvement of the upper parathyroids than the lower ones. The glands are red-brown with foci of cystic change, haemorrhage, and fibrosis. The predominant cell in this form of hyperplasia is the water-clear cell, which is often considerably larger than the normal chief cell (Fig. 93). The cells are filled with multiple small vacuoles which represent dilated Golgi vesicles. The cells contain moderate amounts of glycogen, but stains for neutral lipids are negative. The nuclei are round to ovoid and moderately hyperchromatic, with an eccentrically placed nucleolus. Occasional nuclei may be markedly enlarged and hyperchromatic. Nuclei are often aligned along the vascular pole of the cell, producing a characteristic pattern which has been likened to a bunch of berries. The cells are arranged in large cords and nests. In some instances, the centres of the nests have cystic spaces containing cellular debris.

There is no apparent familial incidence of the disease and no known association with any of the MEN syndromes.

4.4.3 Hyperplasia associated with secondary hyperparathyroidism (Fig. 94)

An increase in parathyroid parenchymal mass resulting from a proliferation of chief cells, oncocytes, and transitional oncocytes in multiple glands in the presence of a known stimulus for parathyroid hormone hypersecretion.

The most common cause of secondary parathyroid hyperplasia is chronic renal failure. Other causes include dietary deficiency of vitamin D, other abnormalities of vitamin D metabolism, and pseudohypoparathyroidism. Once the process of parathyroid hyperplasia begins, the set point for the control of parathyroid hormone secretion by ionic calcium rises, leading to further parathyroid hormone hypersecretion and parathyroid hyperplasia.

The gross appearance of the glands is generally similar to that in patients with primary chief cell hyperplasia; however, there is a greater uniformity of gland size than in patients with primary chief cell hyperplasia. With prolongation of stimulus for parathyroid hormone hypersecretion, there is a tendency to greater variation in gland size.

The earliest change in the glands is a decreased number of fat cells and their replacement by widened cords and nests of chief cells. As the process develops, chief cells may be present in diffuse sheets, cord-like arrangement, follicular patterns, or in trabecular patterns (Fig. 94). Mitotic activity may be evident in some cases. The proliferation of oncocytes may assume nodular configurations and some of the nodules may be surrounded by a fibrous capsule. Foci of adenomatoid change may be prominent in some cases. Although the parathyroid changes that occur in secondary hyperparathyroidism have been classified as hyperplasias, molecular studies indicate that at least some of them may represent clonal proliferations.

Areas of haemorrhage, calcification, chronic inflammation, and cyst formation may be evident, particularly in very large hyperplastic parathyroid glands.

4.4.4   Hyperplasia associated with tertiary hyperparathyroidism

An increase in parathyroid parenchymal mass resulting from a proliferation of chief cells, oncocytes, and transitional oncocytes in multiple glands and resulting in autonomous parathyroid hyperfunction in patients with previously documented, secondary hyperparathyroidism (Table 9).

The histological changes are similar to those described in secondary parathyroid hyperplasia. The predominant cell type is the chief cell, although varying numbers of oncocytes and transitional oncocytes may also be evident. The presence of autonomously functioning clones of chief cells with varying degrees of calcium set point errors may represent the molecular substrates for the development of tertiary hyperparathyroidism.

Adenomas rarely occur in the setting of tertiary hyperparathyroidism.

4.4.5   Cysts

Parathyroid cysts are lined in part by chief cells or contain normal parathyroid tissue within their walls. Cysts may arise from persistent Kursteiner canals, which are found in association with the developing parathyroid. They are uncommon lesions that may present in the cervical region adjacent to the thyroid or in the mediastinum. They are not associated with hyperparathyroidism. Cysts measure from less than 1 cm to more than 10 cm in diameter. The wall of the cyst is composed of fibrous tissue and may include small groups of normal chief cells. The lining of the cyst may contain a layer of flattened chief cells or may be acellular. Cysts containing both thymus and parathyroid are sometimes referred to as third pharyngeal pouch cysts.

Cyst formation may also occur as a result of degenerative changes in adenomas or hyperplasias.

4.4.6   *Parathyromatosis* (Fig. 95)

The presence of hyperplastic aggregates of chief cells in the soft tissues of the neck or mediastinum in patients with primary or secondary parathyroid hyperplasia.

In contrast to invasive parathyroid carcinomas, foci of parathyromatosis lack fibroplasia of the adjacent stroma and do not exhibit evidence of vascular or perineural space invasion. Parathyromatosis may be responsible for persistent or recurrent hyperparathyroidism in patients treated by total parathyroidectomy for primary or secondary hyperplasia.

4.5   Secondary Tumours

Secondary involvement of the parathyroid glands by tumour may occur as a result of direct extension from contiguous structures or by haematogenous or lymphatic spread from distant primary sites. In autopsy series, metastases to the parathyroid glands are found in 12% of patients with disseminated carcinomatosis. The most common sites of origin include breast, skin (melanoma), and lung. Hypoparathyroidism is exceptionally uncommon as a result of secondary involvement of the parathyroid glands by tumour. Rarely, secondary tumours may involve parathyroid adenomas or hyperplastic parathyroid glands.

4.6   Unclassified Tumours

5   Endocrine Tumours of the Pancreas

The endocrine pancreas is composed of (1) the islets of Langerhans, with four cell types, the glucagon (A), insulin (B), somatostatin (D), and pancreatic polypeptide (PP) cells; and (2) single endocrine cells scattered in the exocrine tissue, including (in addition to cells of the above four types) a few serotonin-producing enterochromaffin (EC) cells. Pancreatic endocrine tumours may contain each of these cell types and related hormones, singly or in combination. These tumours may also contain cells not normally found (i.e., ectopic) in the adult human pancreas, e.g., G cells that produce gastrin and cells producing vasoactive intestinal peptide (VIP), growth hormone releasing factor (GRF), adrenocorticotropic hormone (ACTH), and other hor-

Table 10. Clinicopathological correlations of endocrine tumours of the pancreas

1	Well-differentiated endocrine tumour
1.1	Benign behaviour: confined to the pancreas, nonangioinvasive, <2 cm in size[a], ≤2 mitoses and ≤2% Ki67 positive cells/10 HPF
1.1.1	Functioning - insulinoma
1.1.2	Nonfunctioning
1.2	Uncertain behaviour: confined to the pancreas, ≥2 cm in size, >2 mitoses, >2% Ki67 cells/10 HPF, or angioinvasive
1.2.1	Functioning - gastrinoma, insulinoma, vipoma, glucagonoma, somatostatinoma, or inappropriate syndrome[b] tumour
1.2.2	Nonfunctioning
2	Well-differentiated endocrine carcinoma
2.1	Low grade malignant with gross local invasion and/or metastases
2.1.1	Functioning - gastrinoma, insulinoma, glucagonoma, vipoma, somatostatinoma, or inappropriate syndrome[b] tumour
2.1.2	Nonfunctioning
3	Poorly differentiated endocrine carcinoma - small cell carcinoma, high grade malignant

[a] <2 cm in size implies close to 100% probability of benign behaviour, <3 cm corresponds to 90% probability.

[b] Inappropriate hormone syndromes: Cushing (ACTH), acromegaly or gigantism (GRH), hypercalcaemia, etc.

Functioning, associated with pertinent clinical syndrome of endocrine hyperfunction; nonfunctioning, not associated with pertinent clinical syndrome, irrespective of hormone detection in blood or tumour tissue.

mones. The traditional term "islet cell tumour", still sometimes used in the literature, should be restricted to tumours composed only of one or more of the four normal islet cell types. The proposed tumour classification is based largely on the general histological categories recognised for all endocrine tumours (cf Introduction). It additionally includes the specific tumour types identified on the basis of hormone(s) detectable in the tumour and of related hyperfunctional syndrome(s) recognised at the clinical level (Table 10).

5.1   Well-Differentiated Endocrine Tumour (Figs. 96–104)

An epithelial tumour of endocrine cells showing no or minimal atypia and growing in the form of small solid nests, trabeculae, gyriform cords, or, more rarely, pseudoglandular structures.

The individual tumour cells are usually uniform, of small or medium size, with round to oval regular nuclei. There is a variable amount of connective tissue stroma, which may range from highly vascular to collagenised and may exhibit a hyaline appearance. A minority of tumours (mostly insulinomas) contain amyloid. There can be calcification in the stroma, particularly when amyloid is present. The tumours are usually circumscribed, but they may also be ill-defined. Clinically silent microadenomas (0.05 cm–<0.5 cm in size) are found rather frequently in systematic histological investigations at autopsy.

As a rule, tumours confined to the pancreas that are nonangioinvasive, show ≤2 mitoses per 10 high power fields (HPF) and ≤2% Ki-67 positive cells, and are less than 2 cm in diameter follow a benign course (macroadenomas). Tumours confined to the pancreas but showing angioinvasion and/or perineural invasion or >2 mitoses/10 HPF, or >2% Ki-67 positive cells are at increased risk for malignant behaviour. Among the functioning tumours, most insulinomas show benign behaviour, whereas the reverse is true for all the others.

5.2   Well-Differentiated Endocrine Carcinoma
(Figs. 105–110)

A malignant epithelial tumour composed of endocrine cells showing mild to moderate atypia and growing in the form of solid nests and sheets, trabeculae, gyriform cords, or, less commonly, pseudoglandular structures

This tumour shows as signs of malignancy invasion of contiguous structures or documented metastases. Evidence is accumulating that unquestionable angioinvasion and/or perineural space invasion are also an accurate predictor of clinical malignancy. The other histological features of this carcinoma may be indistinguishable from those of well-differentiated endocrine tumours. However, in many cases, the tumour cells have fairly prominent nucleoli in hyperchromatic nuclei, increased numbers of mitoses (2–10 per 10 HPF) and an elevated Ki-67 proliferation index (>5%). Most of these tumours are more than 3 cm in diameter. Metastases, if present, are usually restricted to regional lymph nodes and/or the liver.

5.3   Poorly Differentiated Endocrine Carcinoma – Small Cell Carcinoma (Figs. 111–113)

A malignant epithelial tumour showing highly atypical, small to intermediate sized cells with high nucleocytoplasmic ratio, and poorly granular or agranular cytoplasm, which grows in the form of large, ill-defined solid aggregates, often with central necrosis, and diffuse cellular sheets.

These are highly malignant tumours which, diagnosed as small cell carcinomas, were formerly included among the exocrine tumours of the pancreas. As a rule, the tumours present with distant metastases to the liver and other (often extra-abdominal) sites. Areas of tumour necrosis, >10 mitoses per 10 HPF, >15% Ki-67 positive cells, and prominent angioinvasion or perineural invasion are usually found, frequently combined with P53 protein immunoreactivity.

5.4   Mixed Exocrine-Endocrine Carcinoma (Fig. 114)

An epithelial tumour with a predominant exocrine component admixed with an endocrine component comprising at least one third of the entire tumour cell population.

These are rare tumours, which usually show an intimate admixture of the two components. Their biological behaviour is essentially dictated by the exocrine component, which may be of acinar or ductal type. In the former, the endocrine component is usually composed of islet cell types, while, in the case of ductal endocrine carcinoma, both islet and gut type endocrine cells (especially serotonin and gastrin cells) may be found.

A restricted population of endocrine cells, usually as scattered single cells or forming small aggregates, occurs rather frequently in nonendocrine pancreatic tumours, and it does not influence their clinical behaviour. The only exception is represented by the presence of gastrin cells in mucinous cystadenocarcinomas, which in rare cases have caused Zollinger-Ellison syndrome. Conversely, focal ductal differentiation may occur in otherwise typical islet cell tumours; this rare event should be distinguished from entrapment of normal pancreatic ducts by the tumour growth.

5.5.   Tumour-like Lesions

5.5.1   Islet hyperplasia

An increase in number and size of pancreatic islets, usually resulting from an increase in number and size of beta cells.

Clinically relevant islet hyperplasia has rarely been reported. It has been described in adult patients with α_1-antitrypsin deficiency. In newborns, it has been described in association with maternal diabetes, erythroblastosis fetalis, hereditary tyrosinaemia, and Beckwith-Wiedemann syndrome.

5.5.2   Nesidioblastosis (Fig. 115)

A pancreatic disorder characterised by conspicuously hypertrophic beta cells lying in usually irregularly sized islets and inappropriate insulin secretion.

This is a dysfunctional disease that occurs in newborns or, very rarely, in adults. In familial cases, it is caused by a mutation of the beta cell sulfonylurea-receptor gene and the beta cell ATP-sensitive K^+ channel gene on chromosome 11p15.1. It involves the pancreas diffusely or focally. The disease must be distinguished from simple, clinically irrelevant ductuloinsular complexes, which may be found in the normal newborn pancreas. Rarely, it occurs in the adult pancreas as a result of chronic pancreatitis.

5.5.3   Endocrine dysplasia (Fig. 116)

An endocrine growth less than 0.5 mm in size which deviates from the normal architecture of the islets in having a trabecular structure, abnormal prevalence of one or another of the four islet cell types, and mild cellular atypia.

This lesion has been clearly documented only in the pancreas of patients with type 1 multiple endocrine neoplasia (MEN1).

6   Endocrine Tumours of the Gastrointestinal Tract

Introduction

The normal human gastrointestinal mucosa harbours numerous endocrine cell types. Some of them are restricted to morphologically and functionally well-defined portions of the mucosa, examples being histamine-producing enterochromaffin-like (ECL) cells of gastric acidopeptic glands, gastrin-producing G cells of pyloroduodenal mucosa, and secretin, cholecystokinin (CCK), motilin, or gastric inhibitory polypeptide (GIP) cells of the upper small intestine. Other cells, such as serotonin-producing enterochromaffin (EC) cells or somatostatin D cells, are scattered throughout the entire gastrointestinal tract, while enteroglucagon/PYY-producing L cells and neurotensin cells are present in the lower small intestine, appendix, colon, and rectum.

At present, no or only negligible tumour counterparts have been documented for secretin, CCK, motilin, GIP, and neurotensin cells. Conversely, ECL cells are the main component of gastric endocrine tumours; gastrin and somatostatin cells are a major part of duodenal endocrine tumours; EC cells are the dominant component of endocrine tumours arising in the jejunum, ileum, appendix, and proximal colon (forming the so-called midgut), and enteroglucagon cells predominate among endocrine tumours of the distal colon and rectum (hindgut).

In addition to featuring distinctive cell types, endocrine tumours arising in different parts of the gastrointestinal tract may also show different pathogenetic, histological, and clinical patterns. For practical purposes, it is useful to classify these tumours separately.

The time-honoured term "carcinoid" may be used as synonymous with well-differentiated endocrine tumour of the gut and the term "malignant carcinoid" to designate the corresponding well-differentiated endocrine carcinoma. However, for the sake of clarity, when it comes to clinically functioning tumours, it seems preferable to restrict these terms to tumours associated with the carcinoid syndrome, thus avoiding, for instance, calling a gastrinoma a "carcinoid".

6.1.1   Well-differentiated endocrine tumour – carcinoid

An epithelial tumour of usually monomorphous endocrine cells showing mild or no atypia and growing in the form of solid nests, trabeculae, or pseudoglandulae, restricted to the mucosa or submucosa.

As a rule, the behaviour of nonangioinvasive tumours measuring ≤1 cm in size and showing ≤2 mitoses per 10 HPF is benign. The others are at increased risk of clinical malignancy.

6.1.2   Well-differentiated endocrine carcinoma – malignant carcinoid

A malignant epithelial tumour of endocrine cells showing moderate atypia and growing in the form of solid nests, trabeculae, or larger, less well-defined cellular aggregates, which deeply invades the gut wall (muscularis propria or beyond) or shows metastases to regional lymph nodes or liver.

The tumour is, as a rule, >1 cm in size and may have a moderately elevated mitotic index (>2/10 HPF) or proliferation index (>2% Ki-67 positive cells).

6.1.3   Poorly differentiated endocrine carcinoma – small cell carcinoma

A malignant epithelial tumour composed of highly atypical, small- to intermediate-sized tumour cells growing in the form of large, ill-defined aggregates, often with necrosis and prominent angioinvasion and/or perineural invasion.

The tumour usually shows a highly increased mitotic rate (at least 10/10HPF) and a high proliferation index (>15% Ki-67 positive cells), p53 immunostaining and both local and distant (abdominal and extra-abdominal) metastases.

Endocrine Tumours of the Stomach (Figs. 117–123)

Most endocrine tumours of the stomach are well-differentiated, non-functioning ECL cell tumours (carcinoids) arising in the mucosa of the corpus or fundus. The only well-documented exceptions have been occasional gastrinomas and a few histamine and 5-hydroxytryptophan-producing ECL cell tumours with metastases and the carcinoid syndrome.

ECL cell tumours are often multiple and usually benign. In endoscopic series, most have arisen in a background of diffuse type A (autoimmune, corpus fundus restricted) chronic atrophic gastritis, achlorhydria, and marked hypergastrinaemia, with or without pernicious anaemia. A few cases present in association with hypertrophic-hypersecretory gastropathy with hypergastrinaemia, due to type 1 multiple endocrine neoplasia with Zollinger-Ellison Syndrome (MEN/ZES). Single, often malignant ECL cell tumours also arise at this location, independent of any predisposing mucosal condition. These sporadic tumours are better represented in surgical series. The poorly differentiated small to intermediate cell endocrine carcinomas may arise in any part of the stomach (Table 11).

Table 11. Clinicopathological correlations of endocrine tumours of the stomach

1	Well-differentiated tumour - carcinoid
1.1	Benign behaviour: confined to mucosa-submucosa, nonangioinvasive, ≤ 1 cm in size[a], nonfunctioning
1.1.1	ECL cell tumour of corpus-fundus associated with hypergastrinaemia and chronic atrophic gastritis (CAG) or MEN1 syndrome
1.1.2	Serotonin-producing tumour
1.1.3	Gastrin-producing tumour
1.2	Uncertain behaviour: confined to mucosa-submucosa, >1 cm in size, or angioinvasive
1.2.1	ECL cell tumour with CAG or MEN1 syndrome or sporadic
1.2.2	Serotonin-producing tumour
1.2.3	Gastrin producing tumour
2	Well-differentiated endocrine carcinoma - malignant carcinoid
2.1	Low grade malignant, deeply invasive (muscularis propria or beyond), or with metastasis
2.2	Nonfunctioning
2.2.1	ECL cell carcinoid, usually sporadic, rarely in CAG or MEN1 syndrome
2.2.2	Serotonin-producing carcinoid
2.2.3	Gastrin producing carcinoma
2.3	Functioning
2.3.1	ECL cell carcinoid with atypical carcinoid syndrome
2.3.2	Serotonin-producing carcinoid with carcinoid syndrome
2.3.3	Gastrin-producing carcinoma - malignant gastrinoma
2.3.4	ACTH-producing carcinoma with Cushing syndrome
3	Poorly differentiated endocrine carcinoma - small cell carcinoma, high grade malignant, usually nonfunctioning, occasionally with Cushing syndrome

[a] <1 cm approaches to 100% probability of benign behaviour; <2 cm corresponds to 80% probability

The terms "malignant carcinoid" and "well-differentiated endocrine carcinoma" are essentially equivalent, although the former is traditionally used more for the monoamine-producing EC and ECL cell tumours and the second for the other neoplasms.

Truly mixed exocrine-endocrine carcinomas (with endocrine cells composing more than 30% of the total tumour cell population) are relatively rare in the stomach, despite the frequent occurrence of minor endocrine components in the usual adenocarcinoma. Interestingly, adenomas and adenocarcinomas have been found with some frequency as independent tumours arising in a background of type A chronic atrophic gastritis concomitantly with the more common ECL cell tumours.

Various types of endocrine hyperplasia, from diffuse to linear or micronodular, have been described in the gastric mucosa of hypergastrinaemic subjects with Zollinger-Ellison syndrome or chronic atrophic gastritis. Among these patients, those developing ECL cell tumours (carcinoids) also show dysplastic (precarcinoid) lesions. These are minute (0.15 mm–0.5 mm) nodular growths of mildly atypical cells with a tendency to fuse with each other and invade the lamina propria or develop newly formed stroma.

Endocrine Tumours of the Duodenum and Upper Jejunum
(Figs. 124–126)

The tumours arise mostly in the first and second part of the duodenum and show relevant site-related differences. Nonfunctioning, small gastrin cell tumours confined to the mucosa-submucosa of the proximal duodenal bulb and associated with a benign behaviour are often unexpected findings in gastrectomy or endoscopic specimens. Functioning gastrin cell tumours (gastrinomas) may occur at any site in the duodenum and also in the first jejunal loop. They may be multiple, especially when found in association with the MEN1 syndrome, and very small (a few millimetres), even when metastatic to regional lymph nodes. Occult duodenal microgastrinomas are the likely source of the so-called "primary" lymph node gastrinomas reported in the past (Table 12).

The second portion of the duodenum, especially in and around the papilla and the ampulla, is the preferred site of somatostatin cell tumours, gangliocytic paragangliomas, serotonin-producing EC cell carcinoids, and small cell carcinomas. Somatostatin-producing tumours are often fairly large (several cm in size), deeply invasive,

Table 12. Clinicopathological correlations of endocrine tumours of the duodenum and upper jejunum

1	Well-differentiated endocrine tumour - carcinoid
1.1	Benign behaviour: nonfunctioning, confined to mucosa-submucosa, ≤1 cm in size, nonangioinvasive
1.1.1	Gastrin-producing tumour (proximal duodenum)
1.1.2	Serotonin-producing tumour
1.1.3	Gangliocytic paraganglioma, any size and extension (ampullary region)
1.2	Uncertain behaviour: confined to mucosa-submucosa, >1 cm in size or angioinvasive
1.2.1	Gastrin-producing tumour, functioning (gastrinoma) or nonfunctioning, sporadic, or MEN-1-associated
1.2.2	Somatostatin-producing tumour (ampullary region) with or without Recklinghausen disease
1.2.3	Serotonin-producing tumour, nonfunctioning
2	Well-differentiated endocrine carcinoma - malignant carcinoid
2.1	Low grade malignant: extending beyond submucosa or with metastasis
2.2	Gastrin-producing carcinoma, functioning (gastrinoma) or nonfunctioning, sporadic, or MEN-1-associated
2.3	Somatostatin-producing carcinoma (ampullary region) with or without Recklinghausen disease
2.4	Serotonin-producing carcinoid, nonfunctioning or functioning (any size or extension) with carcinoid syndrome
2.5	Malignant gangliocytic paraganglioma
3.	Poorly differentiated endocrine carcinoma - small cell carcinoma
4	High grade malignant (ampullary region)

and metastatic to regional lymph nodes. They frequently cause obstruction of bile flow and may be associated with neurofibromatosis (Recklinghausen disease), but do not develop the somatostatinoma syndrome found in association with some pancreatic tumours. Due to their microacinar-pseudoglandular structure, the tumours may be misinterpreted as adenocarcinomas, although the occurrence of psammoma bodies should point to the appropriate diagnosis (Table 12).

So-called gangliocytic paragangliomas (a misnomer) are characterised by their dual epithelial endocrine and neuromatous or ganglioneuromatous components. As a rule, they are benign, despite their deep location in the duodenal wall and pseudoinfiltrative patterns of growth. The very few malignant cases have shown metastasis of the epithelial component only (Table 12).

Serotonin-producing EC cell carcinoids are rare, usually nonfunctioning, confined to mucosa-submucosa and benign, whereas the small cell, poorly differentiated carcinomas are highly malignant invasive tumours (Table 12).

Endocrine Tumours of the Ileum, Caecum, Colon, and Rectum
(Figs. 127–129)

Most endocrine tumours of the small intestine and proximal caecum are well-differentiated serotonin and substance-P-producing EC cell tumours (carcinoids), mostly arising in the ileum or distal jejunum. They elicit local obstructive symptoms due to deep invasion, associated with reactive fibrosis. Only a minority of cases, which are metastatic to the liver, cause the typical "carcinoid syndrome" with flushing, blood pressure changes, endocardial fibroelastosis, etc. A few cases have been unexpected, apparently asymptomatic findings in surgical or autopsy specimens. The tumours are frequently multiple and display a distinctive histological structure made up of well-demarcated solid nests with peripheral palisading of highly granular, serotonin-rich tumour cells surrounding an inner part of smaller, less granulated, polyhedral cells (Table 13).

Endocrine tumours of the rectum and sigmoid colon are mainly asymptomatic, small tumours expanding in the submucosa and showing a distinctive trabecular structure. Most tumours produce enteroglucagon or pancreatic polypeptide-related hormones in the absence of a definite hyperfunctional syndrome, although tumour-relat-

Table 13. Clinicopathological correlations of endocrine tumours of the ileum, caecum, colon, and rectum

1	Well-differentiated endocrine tumour - carcinoid
1.1	Benign behaviour: nonfunctioning, confined to mucosa-submucosa, nonangioinvasive, ≤ 1 (small int.) or ≤ 2 cm (large int.) in size
1.1.1	Serotonin-producing tumour
1.1.2	Enteroglucagon-producing tumour
1.2	Uncertain behaviour: nonfunctioning, confined to mucosa-submucosa, >1 cm (small int.) or >2 cm (large int.) in size, or angioinvasive
1.2.1	Serotonin-producing tumour
1.2.1	Enteroglucagon-producing tumour
2	Well-differentiated endocrine carcinoma - malignant carcinoid, low grade malignant, deeply invasive (muscularis propria or beyond), or with metastases
2.1	Serotonin-producing carcinoid with or without carcinoid syndrome
2.2	Enteroglucagon-producing carcinoma
3	Poorly differentiated endocrine carcinoma - small cell carcinoma, high grade malignant
4	Mixed exocrine-endocrine carcinoma - moderate to high grade malignant

ed constipation has occasionally been reported. Serotonin-producing tumours have been observed infrequently in the rectum and distal colon, while enteroglucagon-producing tumours have been found only exceptionally in the small intestine (Table 13).

Highly malignant small cell (poorly differentiated endocrine) carcinomas and mixed mucinous/endocrine carcinomas occur more frequently in the colon and rectum than in the small intestine.

Endocrine Tumours of the Appendix (Fig. 130)

Most carcinoids arise in the deep mucosa and submucosa at the distal tip of the appendix and infiltrate deeply into the wall, causing local symptoms which lead to surgical removal of the tumour. Despite their frequent infiltration of the muscularis propria, most tumours remain confined to the appendix and show benign behaviour. With the exception of a few microtumours, usually 0.5 cm or less in size, composed of enteroglucagon/PYY-producing cells arranged in thin, short trabeculae or tubules, all endocrine tumours of the appendix prove to be serotonin- and substance P-producing EC cell tumours (carcinoids) with a more or less prominent solid nest structure. The few well-differentiated endocrine carcinomas (malignant carcinoids) show invasion of the mesoappendix with or without involvement of the serosa and lymph nodes or distant metastases. Location of the tumour at the base of the appendix, near the caecum, with involvement of the resection margin increases the risk of tumour spread. The car-

Table 14. Clinicopathological correlations of endocrine tumours of the appendix

1	Well-differentiated endocrine tumour - carcinoid, benign behaviour, nonfunctioning, confined to appendiceal wall, nonangioinvasive, ≤2 cm in size
1.1.1	Serotonin-producing tumour
1.1.2	Enteroglucagon-producing tumour - uncertain behaviour, nonfunctioning, confined to subserosa, >2 cm in size, or angioinvasive tumour
2	Well-differentiated endocrine carcinoma - malignant carcinoid
2.1	Low grade malignant, invading the mesoappendix or beyond, and/or with metastasis
2.2	Serotonin-producing carcinoid with or without carcinoid syndrome
3	Mixed exocrine-endocrine carcinoma
3.1	Low grade malignant - goblet-cell carcinoid

cinoid syndrome is observed very rarely and, as a rule, is associated with massive metastases to the liver or retroperitoneum (Table 14).

Small cell carcinoma has not been described in the appendix.

The so-called "goblet cell carcinoid" or "mucocarcinoid" is essentially a low grade adenocarcinoma apparently arising from deep appendiceal crypts (crypt cell carcinoma) and mostly composed of clusters of mucin-containing cells with scattered endocrine cells. Only occasionally is the proportion of endocrine cells (mainly serotonin-containing EC cells) in the tumour large enough to justify its diagnosis as a mixed endocrine-exocrine tumour (Table 14).

Multiple Endocrine Neoplasia Type 1

Multiple endocrine neoplasia type 1 (MEN1) is an endocrine disorder inherited as an autosomal dominant trait and characterised by the development of endocrine tumours mainly involving the anterior pituitary, parathyroids, endocrine pancreas, and duodenum.

A variety of germline mutations of the MEN1 gene located on chromosome 11q13 have been associated with the disease. In MEN1, multiple endocrine tumours arise in the pancreas and duodenum, in the parathyroids, and in the pituitary. In addition to these lesions, endocrine tumours may develop (in descending order of frequency) in the thymus, lung, stomach, and jejunum-ileum. Their incidence ranges from 5% to 9%. Adrenocortical, lipomatous, and thyroid lesions may also occur.

Parathyroid glands. The parathyroid glands of MEN patients show diffuse or nodular proliferations of chief cells, often admixed with some oncocytic cells. All parathyroid glands are usually involved, but an asymmetric and mainly nodular enlargement of the parathyroid glands with at least one normal-sized gland present may occur in half of the individuals. The parathyroid changes are generally referred to as hyperplasia. However, it is difficult or even impossible to distinguish the parathyroid lesions in MEN1 from sporadic adenomas. In addition, there have been single reports describing the occurrence of parathyroid carcinoma.

Pancreas. The outstanding histological feature of the pancreatic lesions is the presence of numerous microadenomas spread throughout the pancreas, together with occasional larger tumours (macrotumours) with diameters greater than 0.5 cm. The total number of tumours in a pancreas may vary considerably among MEN1 patients. The small tumours usually display a distinct trabecular pattern and may show conspicuous connective tissue stroma. The larger tumours may show a solid or trabecular histological pattern. If one of these tumours exhibits amyloid deposition, it is usually associated with insulin production. Immunocytochemically, the tumours consistently express multiple hormones, with one hormone usually prevailing. Pancreatic polypeptide- and glucagon-containing tumours are most often found, while tumours expressing insulin predominantly or exclusively are less common; and gastrin-producing tumours are relatively uncommon. The pancreatic tumours only rarely give rise to metastases.

In contrast to earlier assumptions, nesidioblastosis and islet hyperplasia are not a feature of the MEN1 pancreas. The latter change is only seen in cases with additional severe obstructive pancreatitis due to duct stenosis caused by large endocrine tumours. Nesidioblastosis with islet hyperplasia cannot therefore be regarded as the precursor lesion of the pancreatic tumours in MEN1. Instead, the pancreatic tumours appear to originate directly from islets.

Duodenum. The duodenum, like the pancreas, harbours multiple, tiny endocrine tumours (<1 cm) in the mucosa and submucosa. They most often reside in the proximal duodenum. Immunocytochemically, these tumours stain almost exclusively for gastrin. Periduodenal-parapancreatic lymph node metastases are found in up to 80% of the cases and may be much larger than the primary tumour. The development of liver metastases is rare and occurs late in the course of the disease.

Pituitary. The anterior pituitary gland usually contains a single tumour, but multicentricity has also been reported. Immunocytochemically, most tumours produce GH and/or PRL and only occasionally stain for ACTH. Diffuse hyperplasia of one of the cell types has not yet been recorded.

Stomach. The stomach of MEN1 patients with Zollinger-Ellison syndrome shows diffuse hyperplasia of ECL cells in the corpus fundus mucosa. In addition, there may be multiple ECL (argyrophil endocrine) tumours (carcinoids), which are often of considerable size, but only rarely associated with metastases.

Thymus and Lung. The endocrine tumours that occur in the thymus may show invasion and/or metastasis at the time of diagnosis. Many stain for ACTH. The lung tumours are usually small and correspond to well-differentiated endocrine tumours (typical carcinoids).

Adrenal glands. The changes in the adrenal cortex include diffuse and nodular hyperplasia and multiple adenomas. Most of these lesions are nonfunctioning. Adrenal carcinomas are rare.

Clinicopathological features. The most common hyperfunctional syndrome is hyperparathyroidism (due to parathyroid lesions), followed by Zollinger-Ellison syndrome (due to duodenal or pancreatic tumours), hyperinsulinaemic syndrome (due to pancreatic tumours), prolactinoma syndrome (due to pituitary tumours), Cushing syndrome (due to pituitary or thymic tumours), growth-hormone-releasing-factor-induced acromegaly, vipoma, and glucagonoma syndrome (due to pancreatic tumours). Loss of heterozygosity at site q13 on chromosome 11 is usually found in tumour tissue. Analysis for a germline mutation of the MEN1 gene can be done on blood cells of the proband and his relatives.

Multiple Endocrine Neoplasia Type 2

Multiple endocrine neoplasia type 2 (MEN2) is an endocrine disorder inherited as an autosomal dominant trait. There are three variants, which share medullary thyroid carcinoma as part of the disease: MEN2A, or Sipple syndrome, is characterised by the development of medullary thyroid carcinoma, pheochromocytoma, and parathyroid hyperplasia; MEN2B is characterised by the development of medullary thyroid carcinoma and pheochromocytoma in association with gastrointestinal ganglioneuromatosis, a marfanoid habitus, and other occasional lesions such as parathyroid hyperplasia and a variety of skeletal abnormalities; familial medullary thyroid carcinoma (FMTC) is characterised by the development of medullary thyroid carcinoma in at least four family members.

All three variants are caused by germline mutations in the *RET* proto-oncogene located on chromosome 10q11.2. MEN2A accounts for more than 90%, and MEN2B for approximately 5% of all MEN2 patients.

Thyroid C cells. MEN2-associated medullary thyroid carcinoma is usually multifocal and bilateral. Most frequently, it is located in the middle or upper part of the thyroid lobes. The histological pattern, cytological features, and metastatic spread are similar to those of sporadic medullary thyroid carcinoma. MEN2-associated medullary thyroid carcinoma is preceded by bilateral and multicentric C cell hyperplasia, which is defined as the presence of a minimum of 50 C cells (or 40 cells per cm^2) in at least three low power fields. As C cell hyperplasia in MEN 2 progresses to medullary thyroid carcinoma, C cells replace the follicular epithelium (diffuse C cell hyperplasia) and produce small intrafollicular nodules (nodular C cell hyperplasia). Transition from nodular C cell hyperplasia to microscopic medullary thyroid carcinoma occurs when C cells are found to invade through the follicular basement membrane into the thyroid stroma, leading to a stromal reaction.

Adrenal medulla. MEN2 associated pheochromocytoma is usually multicentric and bilateral. Otherwise, it does not differ from sporadic pheochromocytoma. MEN2-associated pheochromocytoma is preceded by diffuse or nodular adrenal medullary hyperplasia, which is defined as the enlargement of the adrenal medulla beyond the normal cortex/medulla ratio of 10:1. Nodules larger than 1 cm in diameter are considered pheochromocytomas, while smaller nodules are defined as nodular medullary hyperplasia. MEN2-associated pheochromocytoma has not been found to be associated with malignant behaviour.

Parathyroid lesions. Diffuse or nodular (chief cell) hyperplasia of the parathyroid glands occurs in approximately 70% of MEN2A patients and 20% of MEN2B patients. Occasionally, parathyroid adenomas occur in combination with the hyperplastic changes.

Ganglioneuromatosis. Ganglioneuromatosis is a feature of MEN2B. It is characterised by the proliferation of nerves, ganglion, and Schwann cells in the submucosal and intramuscular plexuses. It involves the mucosa of the upper aerodigestive tract, the lips and tongue, and the gastrointestinal tract.

Associated lesions. Skeletal abnormalities resulting in a marfanoid habitus are features of MEN2B. Other occasional associated lesions include skin amyloidosis (so-called cutaneous lichen amyloidosis), which is usually located in the interscapular region, and Hirschsprung disease.

Clinicopathological features. Only 40% of MEN2 patients exhibit the "classical" sequence of the disease, in which they first develop medullary thyroid carcinoma followed by pheochromocytoma causing hypertension due to excess catecholamine secretion. In MEN2A, 20% of these patients develop overt hyperparathyroidism. In MEN2B, gastrointestinal ganglioneuromatosis is accompanied by constipation or diarrhoea. Approximately 25%–30% of these patients develop megacolon or, more rarely, diverticulosis. MEN2A, MEN2B, and FMTC are caused by germline mutations in the RET proto-oncogene, which is localised on chromosome 10q11.2.

Ectopic Hormone Production

The term "ectopic hormone" indicates a tumour-produced hormone that is not normally produced by the tissue from which the tumour originates.

The precise histological classification of tumours producing ectopic hormones and their correlation with pertinent clinical syndromes is important. Significant associations have been observed between particular tumour histotypes and production of specific hormones. Most tumours producing ectopic hormones prove to be malignant, ranging from low grade, well-differentiated endocrine carcinomas to high grade small cell carcinomas. Clinical syndromes are much less frequent than mere hormone production by tumour cells. Table 15 lists the more frequently involved tumour types, along with the hormones produced and the pertinent clinical syndromes.

Table 15. Ectopic hormones, main tumour sources, and related syndromes

Hormone	Tumour type	Clinical syndrome[a]
Hypothalamic and neurohypophyseal hormones		
Antidiuretic hormone (ADH)	Lung carcinoma (small cell) and pancreatic adenocarcinoma, adrenal carcinoma	Syndrome of inappropriate antidiuretic hormone
Oxytocin	Lung carcinoma (small cell)	
Corticotropin-releasing hormone (CRH)	Lung carcinoma (small cell), pancreatic endocrine carcinoma	Cushing syndrome
Thyrotropin-releasing hormone (TRH)	Lung carcinoma (small cell)	
Growth-hormone-releasing hormone	Bronchial carcinoid, pancreatic endocrine tumours	Acromegaly
Adenohypophyseal hormones		
ACTH	Lung carcinoma (small cell) and carcinoid, pancreatic endocrine carcinoma, thyroid medullary carcinoma, pheochromocytoma, thymus carcinoid	Cushing syndrome
Prolactin	Lung carcinoma, renal carcinoma	Galactorrhea
GH	Lung carcinoma	Acromegaly
Gonadotropins	Lung carcinoma	
Thyrotropin	Trophoblastic disease	Thyrotoxicosis
Gastroenteropancreatic hormones		
Insulin	Gastric carcinoma, lung carcinoma	Hypoglycaemia
Insulin-like growth factors I-II (IGF I-II)	Sarcomas, hepatocellular carcinoma	Hypoglycaemia
Gastrin releasing peptide (GRP, bombesin)	Lung carcinoma (small cell) and carcinoid	
Gastrin	Pancreatic endocrine tumours, mucinous cystic tumours of the ovary or pancreas	Zollinger-Ellison syndrome
Vasoactive intestinal peptide (VIP)	Pancreatic endocrine tumours	Verner-Morrison syndrome
Somatostatin	Lung carcinoma (small cell) and carcinoid, pheochromocytoma	

---

[a] Clinical syndromes are usually much less frequent than hormone productions.

Table 15 *(continued)*

Hormone	Tumour type	Clinical syndrome[a]
Various hormones		
Human chorionic gonadotropin (hCG)	Trophoblastic disease, ovarian and testicular tumours, carcinomas of different sites	Gynaecomastia/ loss of libido
Calcitonin	Well and poorly differentiated endocrine carcinomas of various sites (lung, pancreas, etc.), pheochromocytoma	
Parathyroid hormone (parathyrin)	Lung carcinoma, pancreatic endocrine carcinoma, uterine carcinoma, ovarian carcinoma	Hypercalcaemia
Parathyroid hormone-related peptide (PTHRP)	Lung carcinoma (squamous), hepatocellular carcinoma	Hypercalcaemia
Erythropoietin	Renal carcinoma, uterine leiomyoma	Erythrocytosis

[a] Clinical syndromes are usually much less frequent than hormone productions.

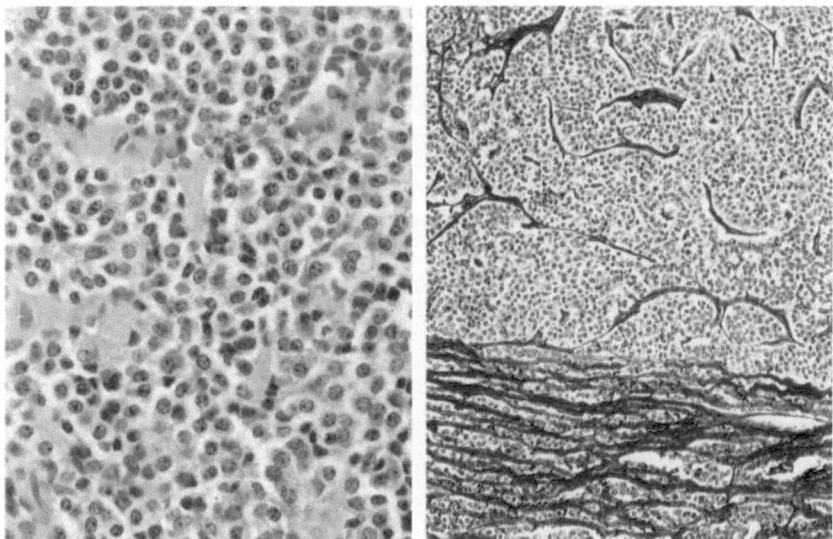

Fig. 1. Pituitary adenoma. *Left* Benign cytology with inconspicuous nucleoli and diagnostic loss of the acinar pattern as well as *right* compression of adjacent normal parenchyma. (Gomori reticulin)

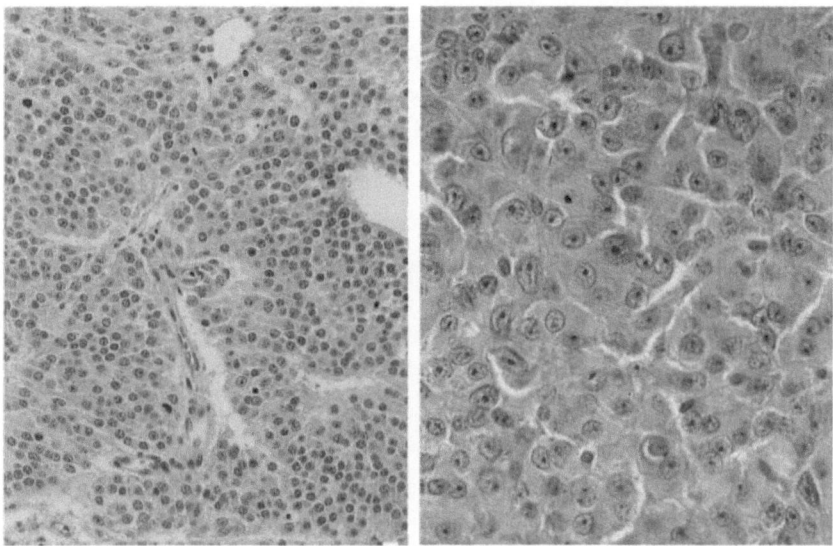

Fig. 2. Atypical pituitary adenoma. *Left* Variable mitotic activity and *right* nucleolar prominence

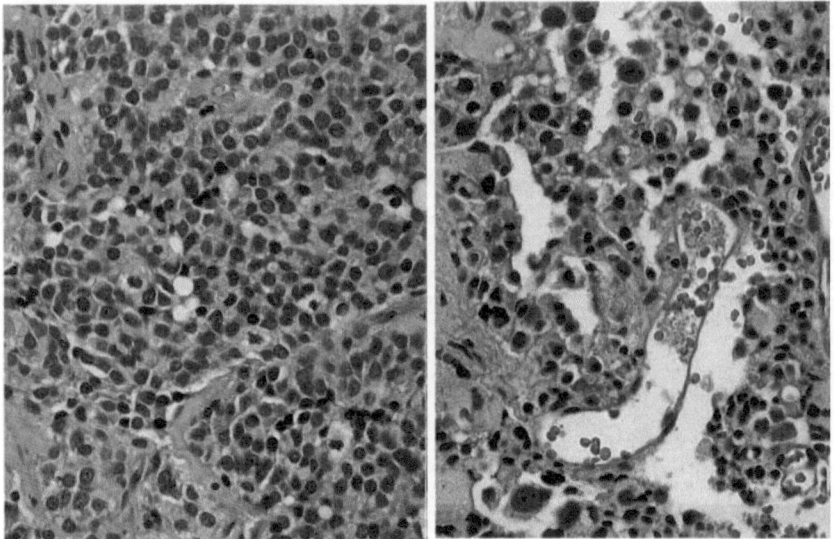

Fig. 3. Pituitary carcinoma. *Left* Some tumours feature mitotic activity but lack obvious cytological atypia, whereas *right* others showing marked cytological atypia may be unassociated with significant mitotic activity

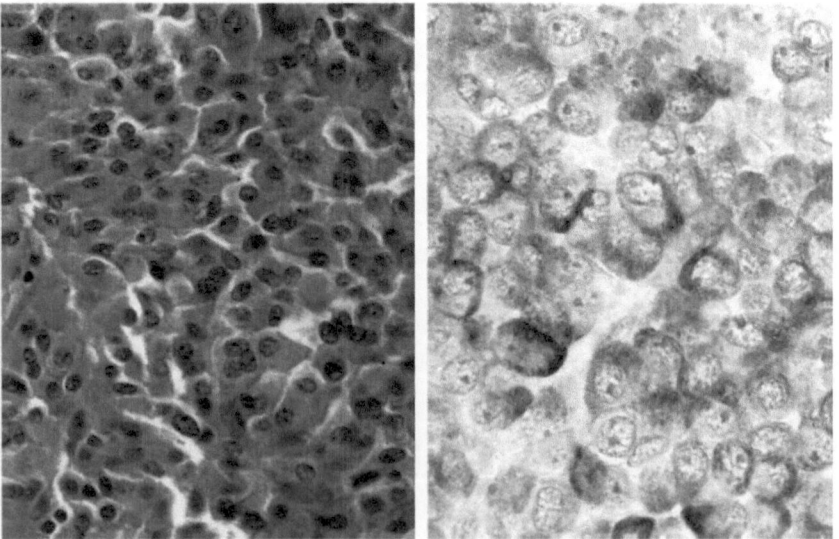

Fig. 4. Densely granulated GH cell adenoma. *Left* H&E. *Right* GH immunostain

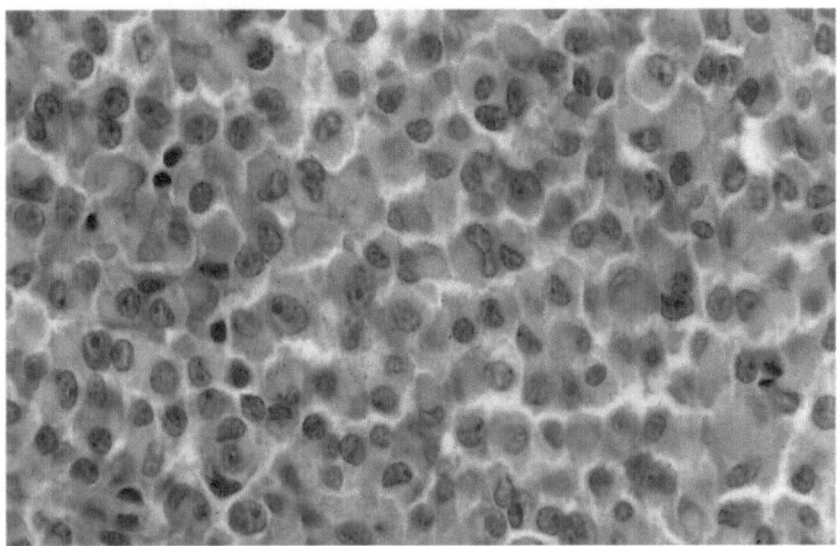

Fig. 5. Sparsely granulated GH cell adenoma. Cytoplasmic fibrous bodies

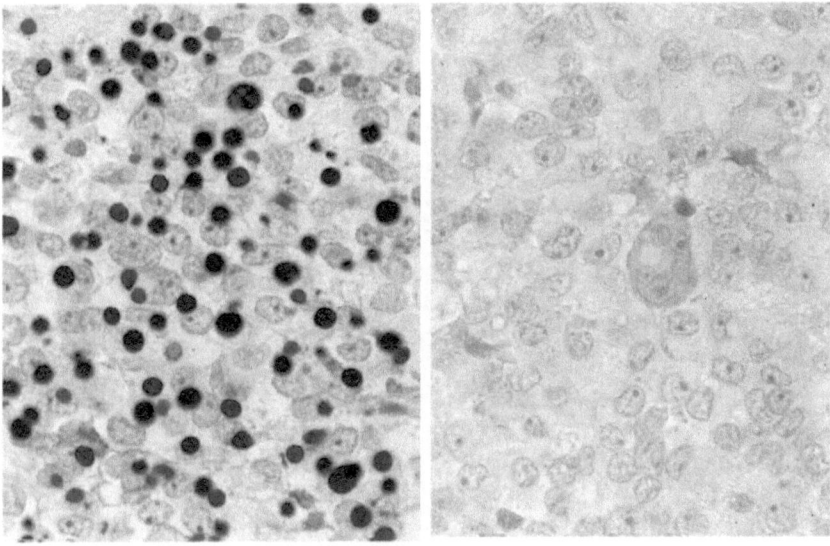

Fig. 6. Sparsely granulated GH cell adenoma. *Left* Fibrous bodies are immunoreactive for keratin. *Right* GH immunoreactivity is often sparse

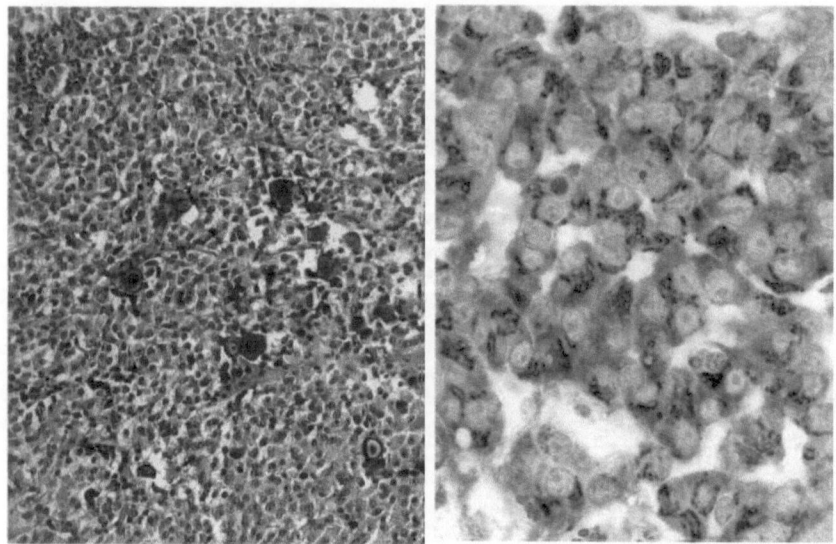

Fig. 7. Prolactin cell adenoma. *Left* Microcalcifications in the chromophobic tumour. *Right* Immunostain for PRL showing Golgi pattern reactivity

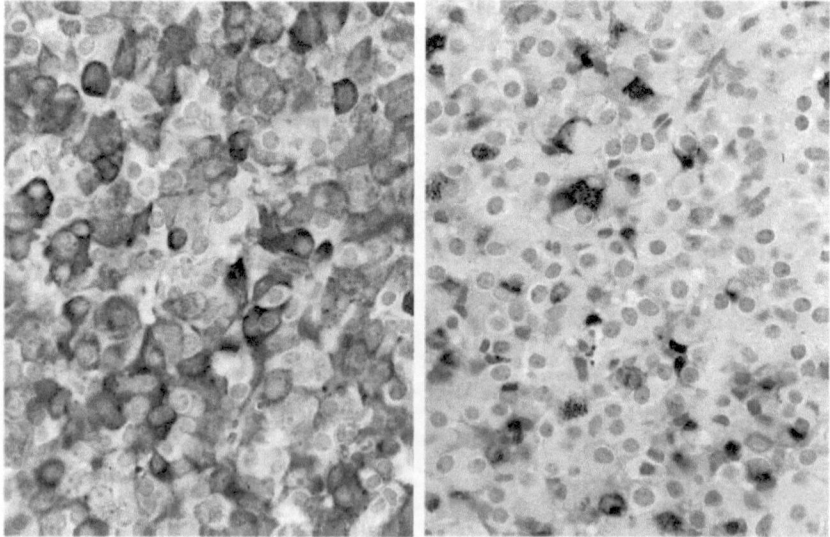

Fig. 8. Mixed GH cell – PRL cell adenoma. *Left* GH immunostain and *right* PRL immunostain

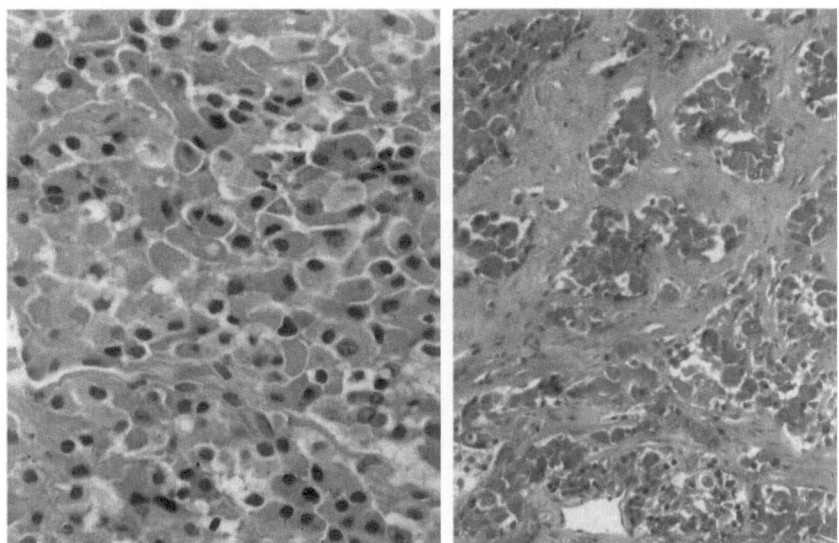

Fig. 9. ACTH cell adenoma. *Left* Amphophilia. *Right* Stromal fibrosis, an uncommon feature

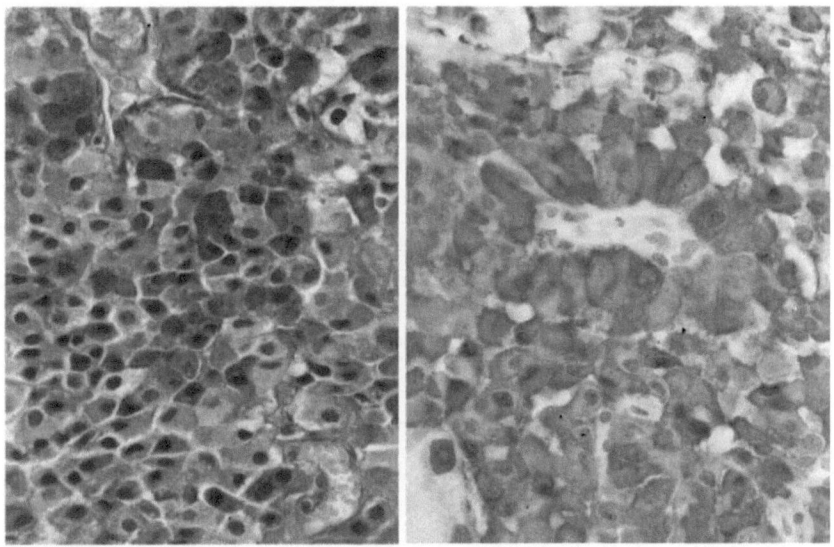

Fig. 10. ACTH cell adenoma. *Left* PAS staining. *Right* ACTH immunoreactivity

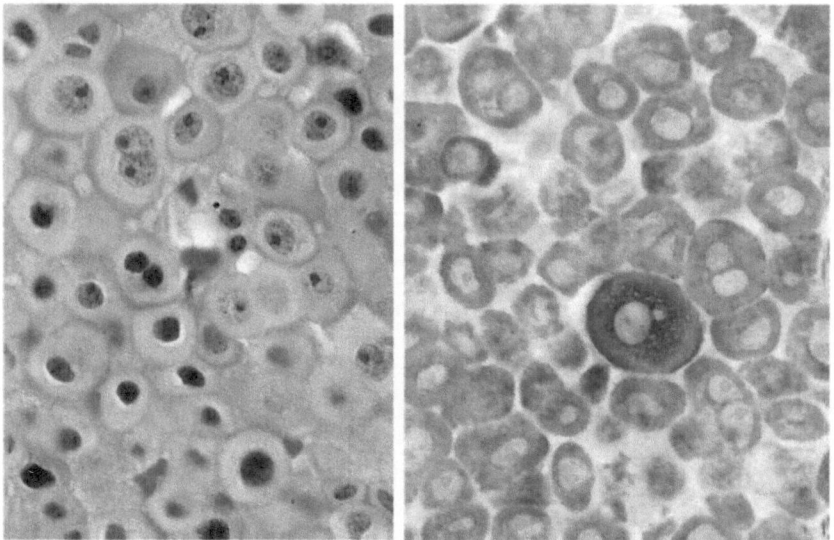

Fig. 11. Crooke cell adenoma. *Left* H&E. *Right* Keratin immunostain

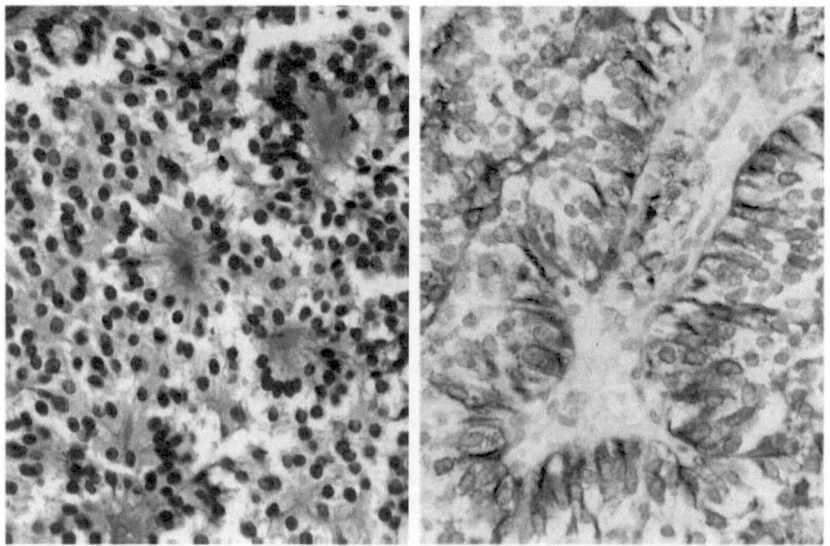

Fig. 12. LH/FSH adenoma. *Left* Papilla formation. *Right* Immunostain for LH

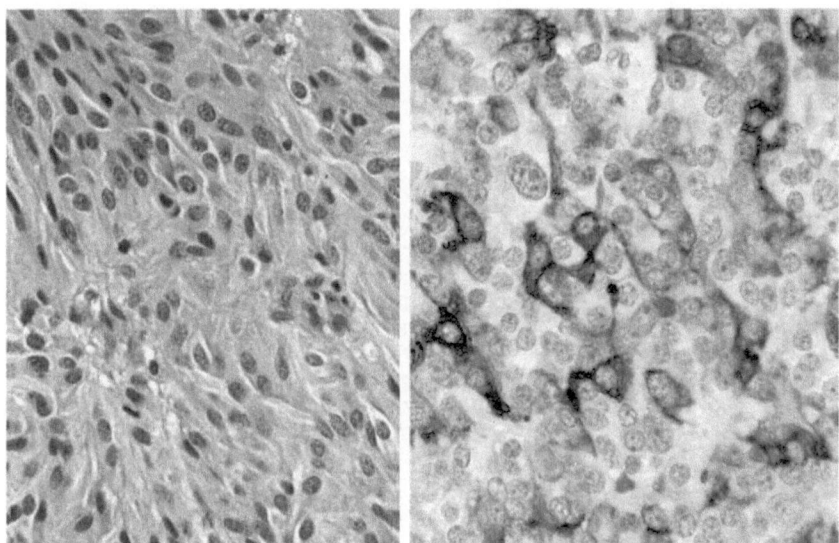

Fig. 13. TSH cell adenoma. *Left* Elongate cells. *Right* TSH immunostain

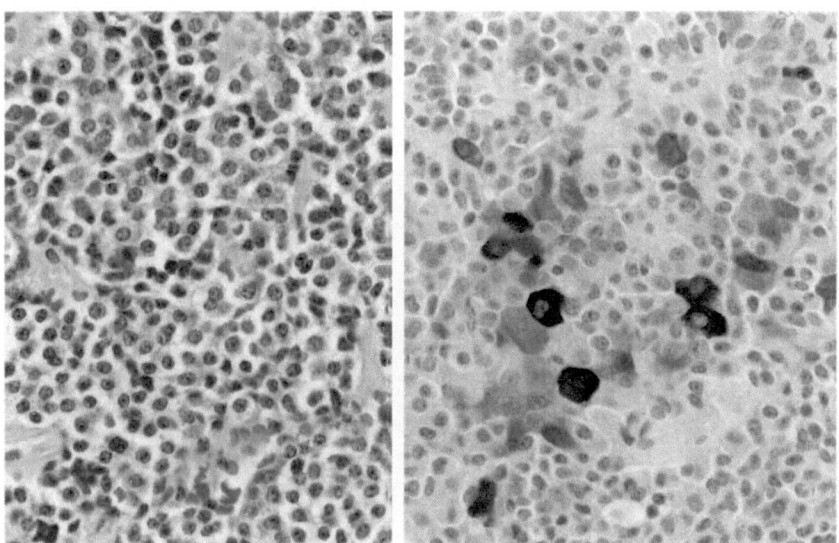

Fig. 14. Null cell adenoma, nononcocytic type. *Left* H&E. *Right* Immunostain for alpha subunit

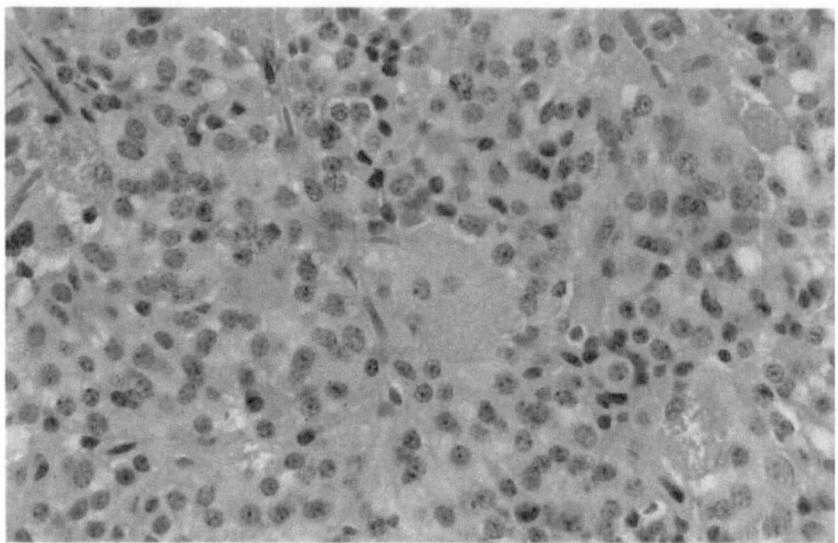

Fig. 15. *Null cell adenoma, oncocytic type*

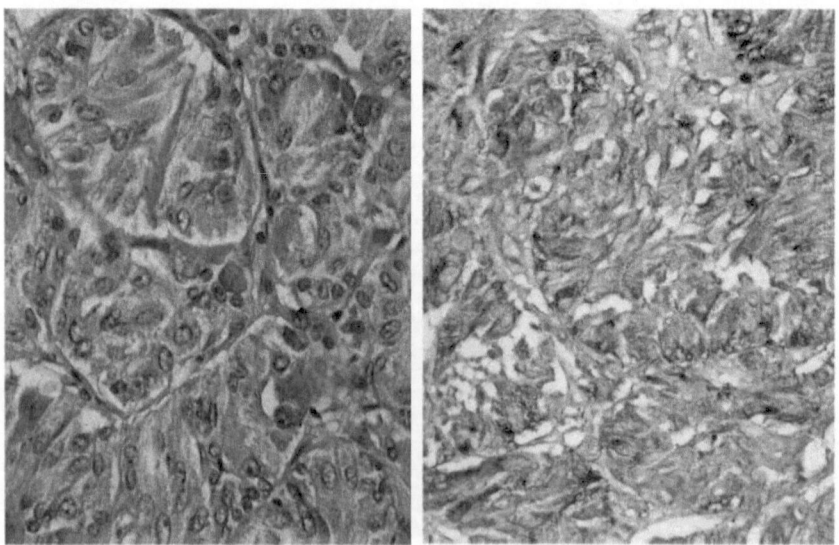

Fig. 16. *Pituitary hyperplasia. TSH cell hyperplasia in hypothyroidism. Left* Expanded acini composed of uniform, elongate TSH cells. *Right* TSH immunostain

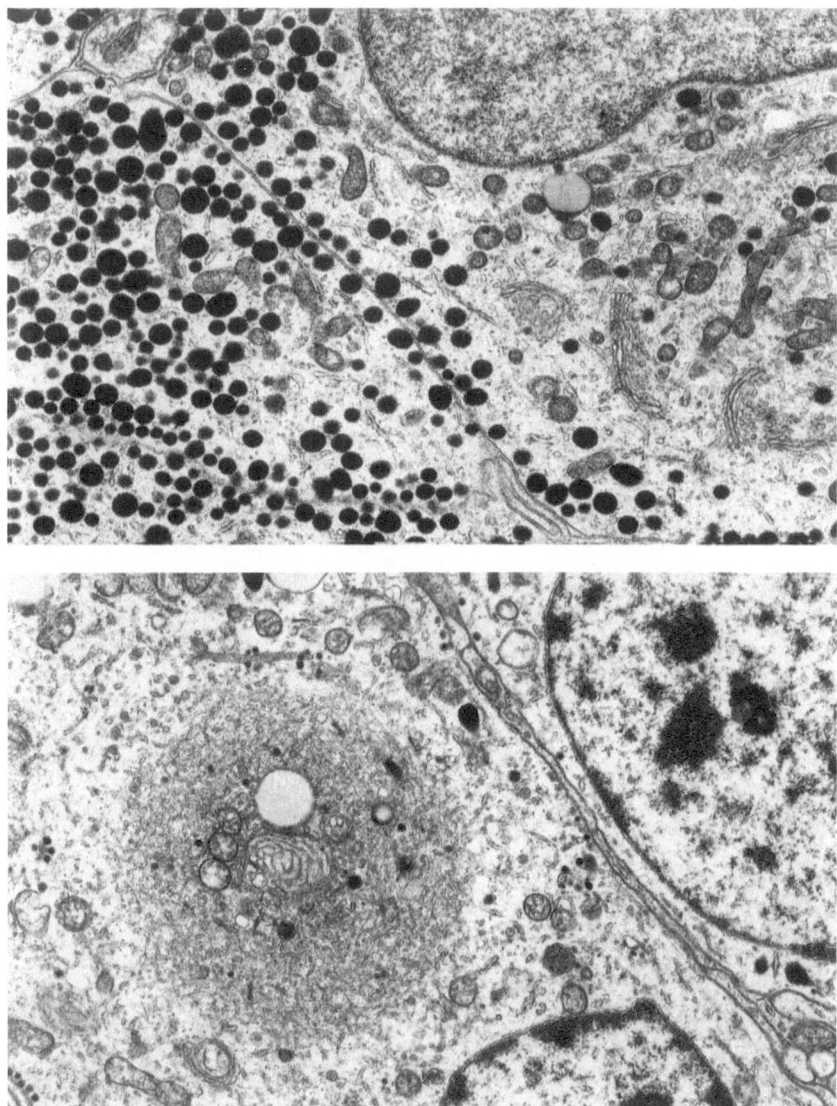

Fig. 17. *Top* Densely granulated GH cell adenoma, x 10,500. *Bottom* Sparsely granulated GH cell adenoma with fibrous body. x 9,250

84

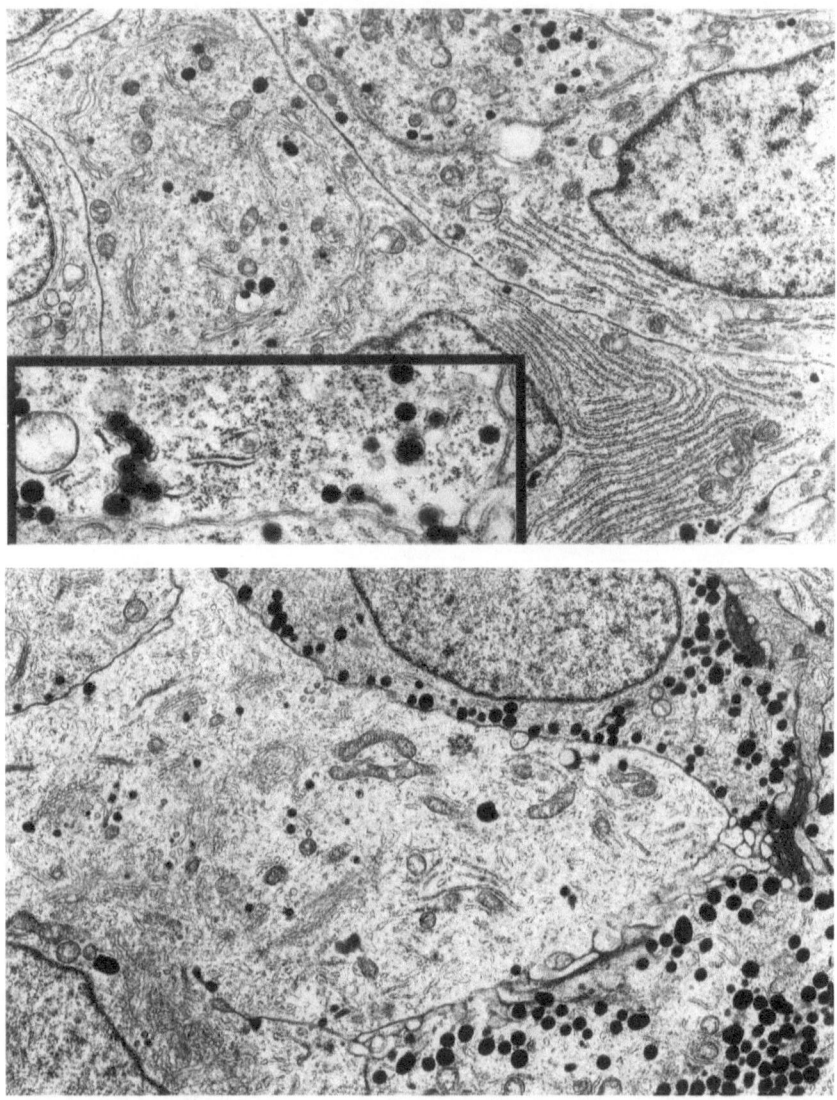

Fig. 18. *Top* Prolactin cell adenoma, x 6,600. *Inset* Note "misplaced exocytoses", x 17,750. *Bottom* Mixed GH cell and PRL cell adenoma, showing densely granulated GH cells and sparsely granulated PRL cells, x 8,700

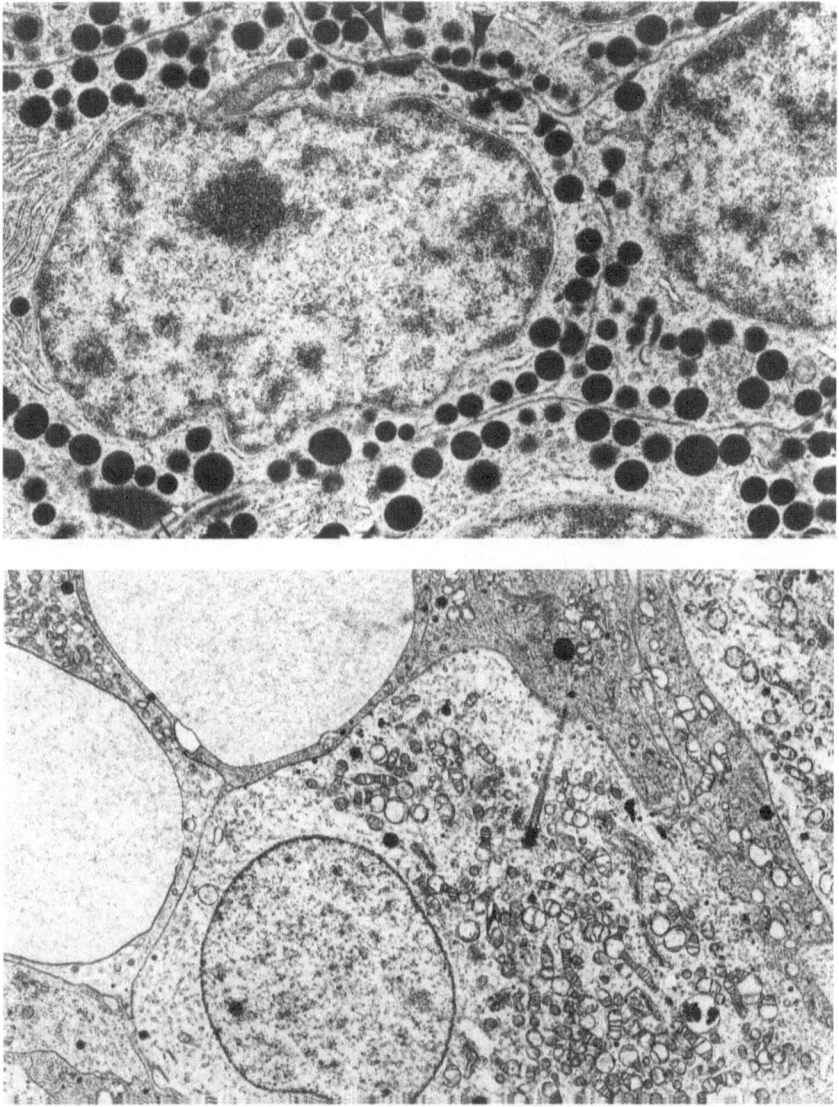

Fig. 19. *Top* Mammosomatotroph cell adenoma. Large granules and extracellular deposits of secretory material (*arrowheads*), x 11,000. *Bottom* Acidophil stem cell adenoma with giant spherical mitochondria in the lower right part, x 4,480

86

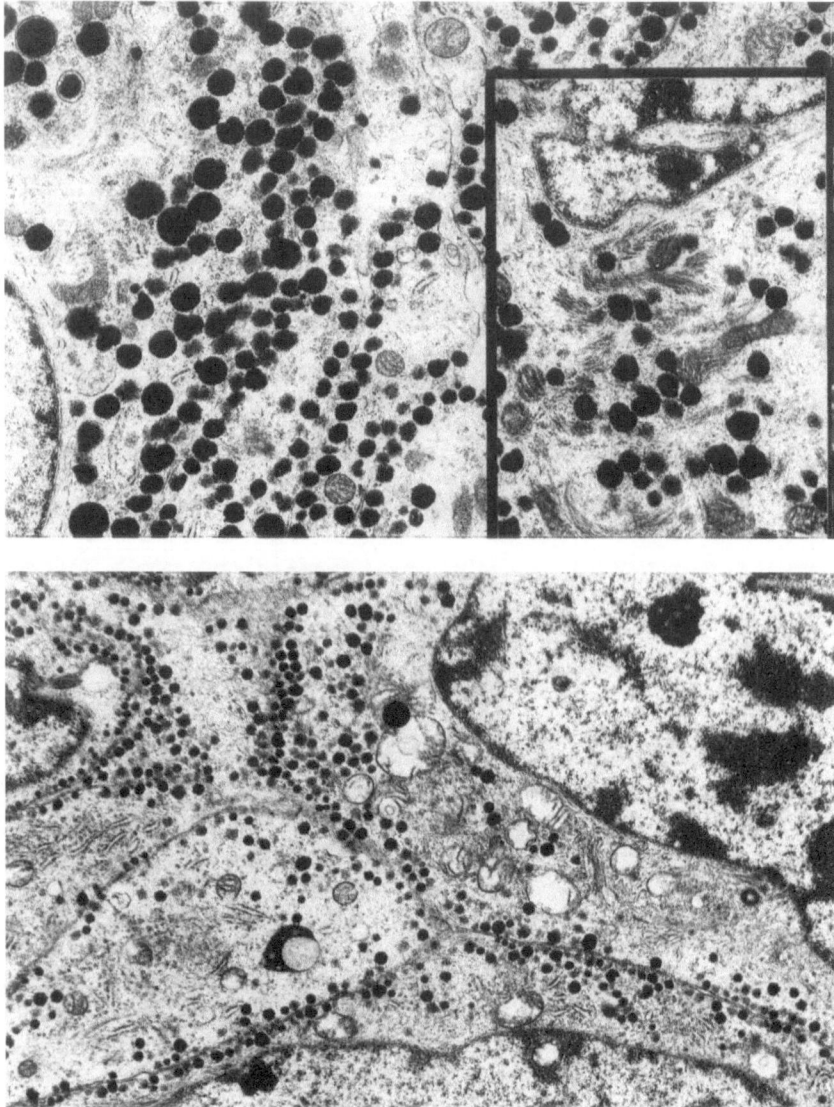

Fig. 20. *Top* ACTH cell adenoma, x 11,440. *Inset,* x 13,200, shows intermediate filament (cytokeratin) bundles. *Bottom* Sparsely granulated ACTH cell adenoma. Occasional indented or heart-shaped secretory granules and intermediate filament (cytokeratin) bundles are present, x 9,070

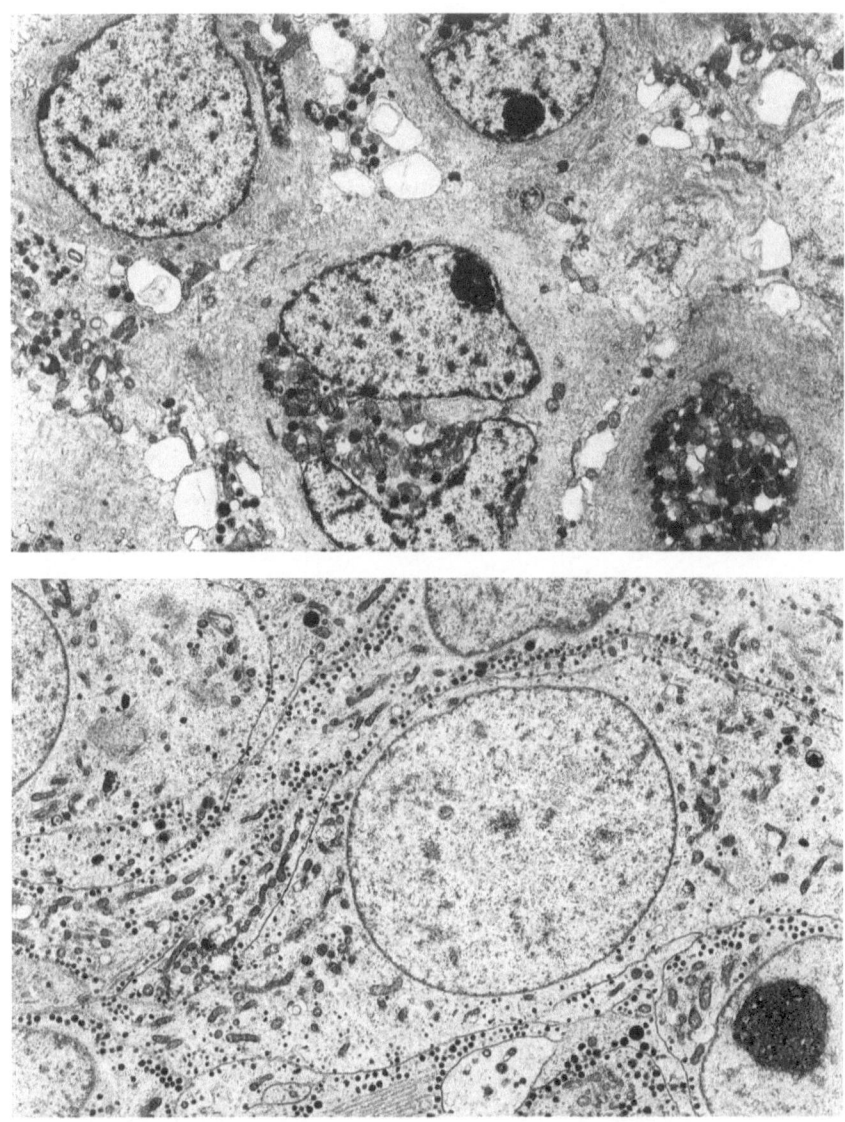

Fig. 21. *Top* Crooke cell adenoma, x 4,640. *Bottom* TSH cell adenoma, x 4,160

88

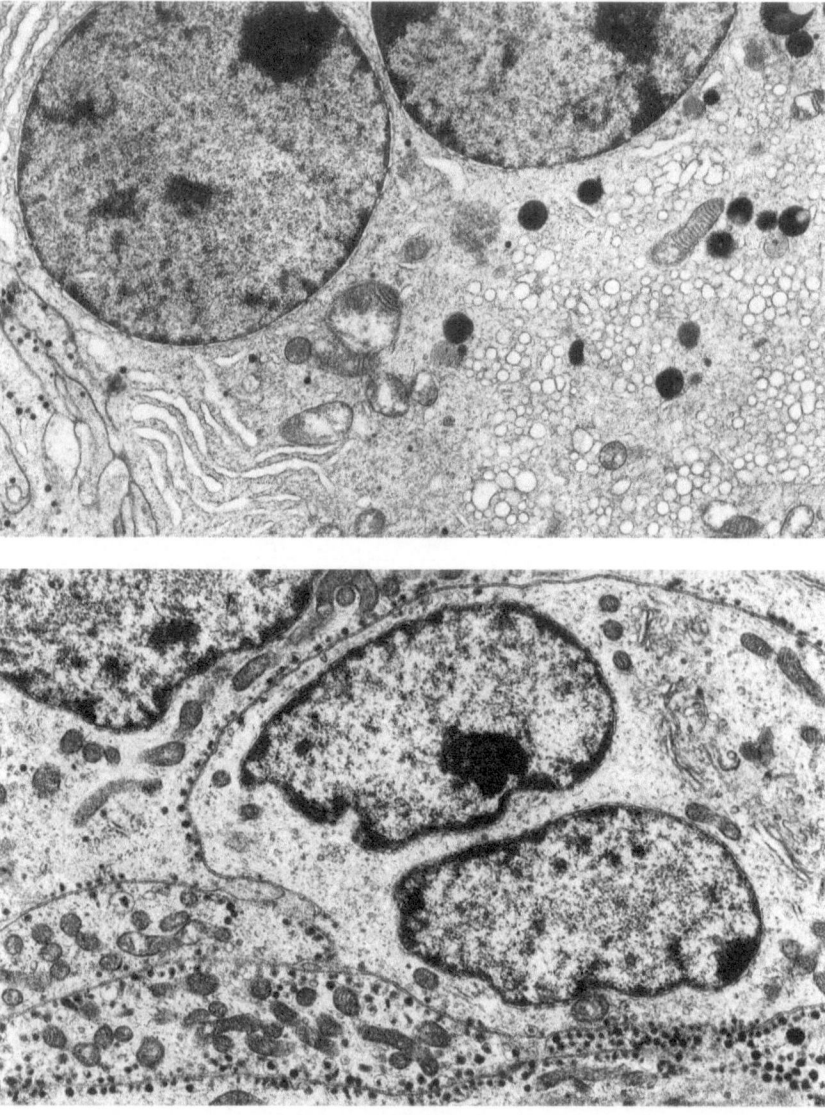

Fig. 22. *Top* LH/FSH adenoma, "female type", x 8,100. Note vacuolar or "honey-comb" transformation of the Golgi complex. *Bottom* LH/FSH adenoma, "male type", x 10,120

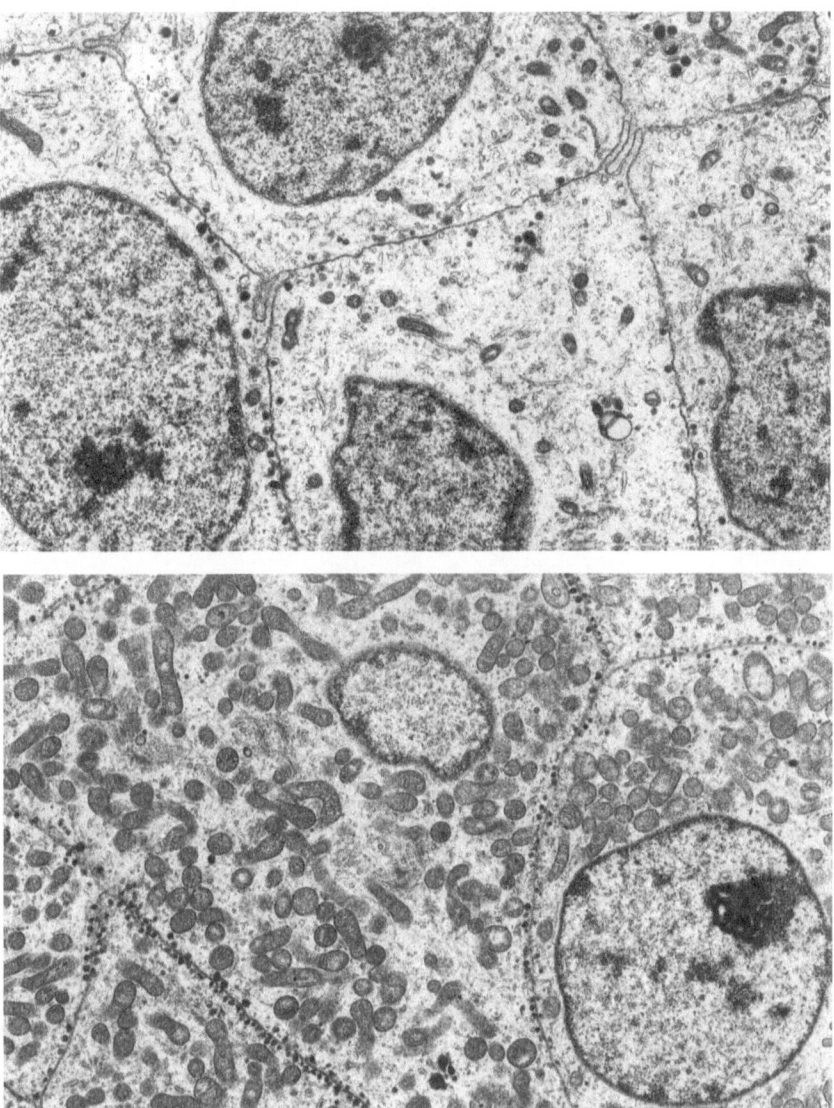

Fig. 23. *Top* Null cell adenoma, nononcocytic type, x 6,960. *Bottom* Null cell adenoma, oncocytic type, x 5,500

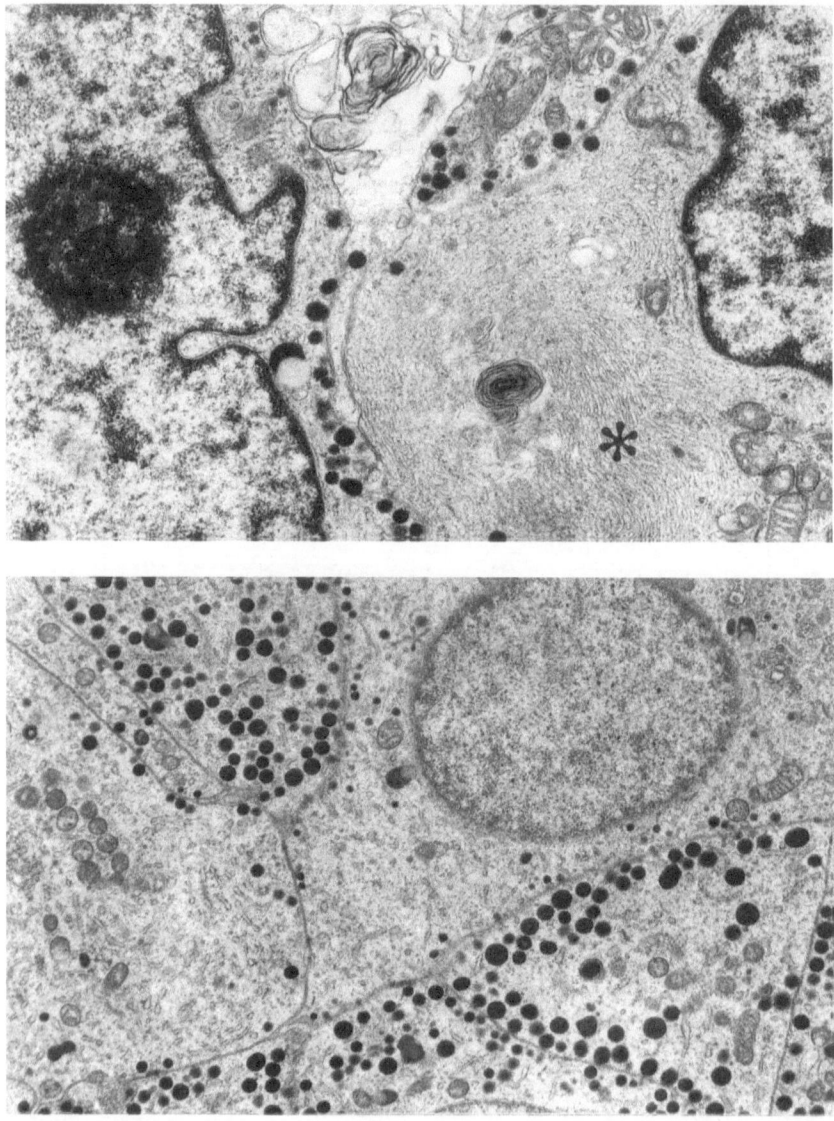

Fig. 24. *Top* Silent "corticotroph" cell adenoma, subtype 3, x 12,650. Note abundance of smooth endoplasmic reticulum *(asterix)*. x 7,500. *Bottom* Plurimorphous adenoma composed of densely granulated GH cells as well as TSH cells, x 7,400

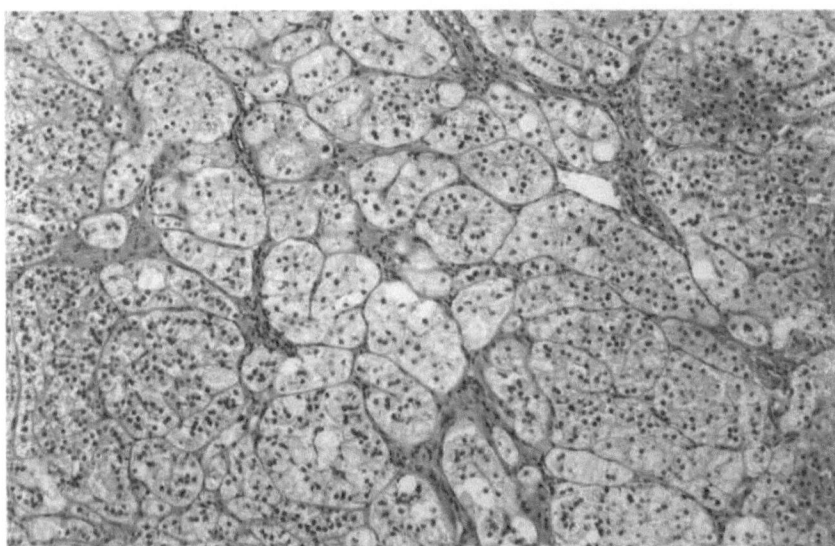

Fig. 25. Adrenal cortical adenoma with hypercortisolism (Cushing syndrome). Tumour is composed of cells with pale-staining, lipid-rich cytoplasm with predominantly alveolar or nesting pattern. Short blunt cords are also present

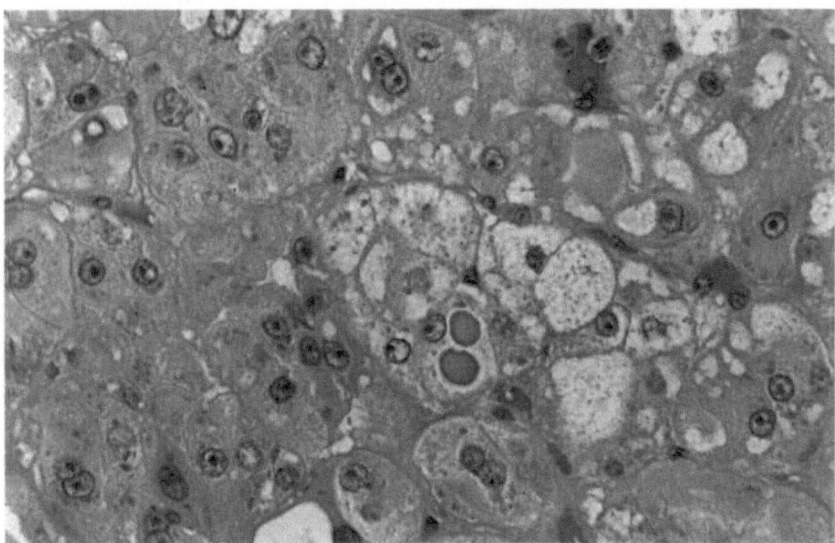

Fig. 26. Adrenal cortical adenoma with Cushing syndrome. There is a mixture of cells arranged in a predominantly trabecular pattern with compact eosinophilic and lipid-rich cytoplasm. Nuclei are somewhat vesicular with a small, dot-like nucleolus. Note the few intracytoplasmic hyaline globules near centre of field

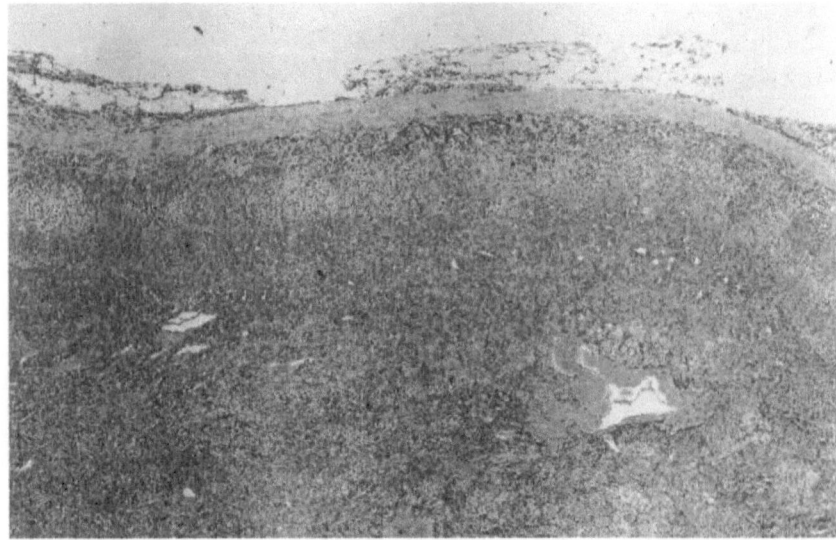

Fig. 27. Adrenal cortical adenoma with Cushing syndrome. Marked atrophy of adjacent cortex due to suppression of ACTH secretion

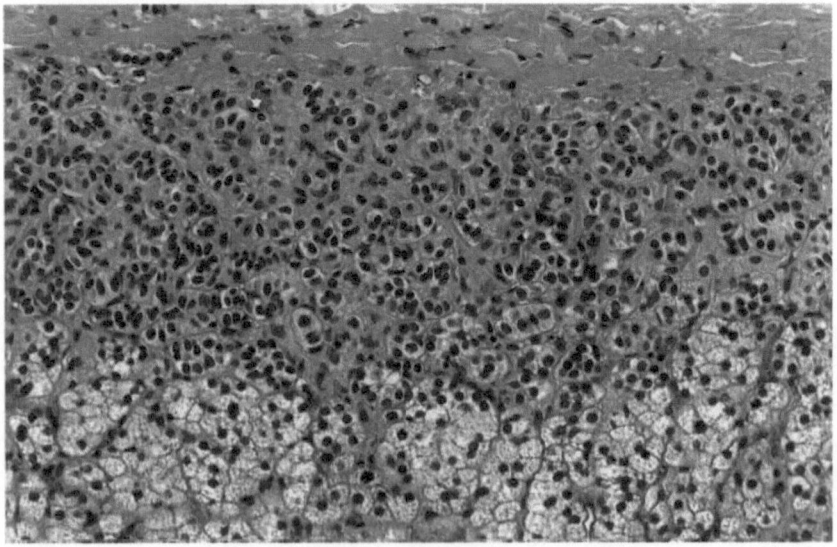

Fig. 28. Adrenal cortical adenoma with primary hyperaldosteronism (Conn syndrome). Adrenal remnant shows hyperplasia of zona glomerulosa

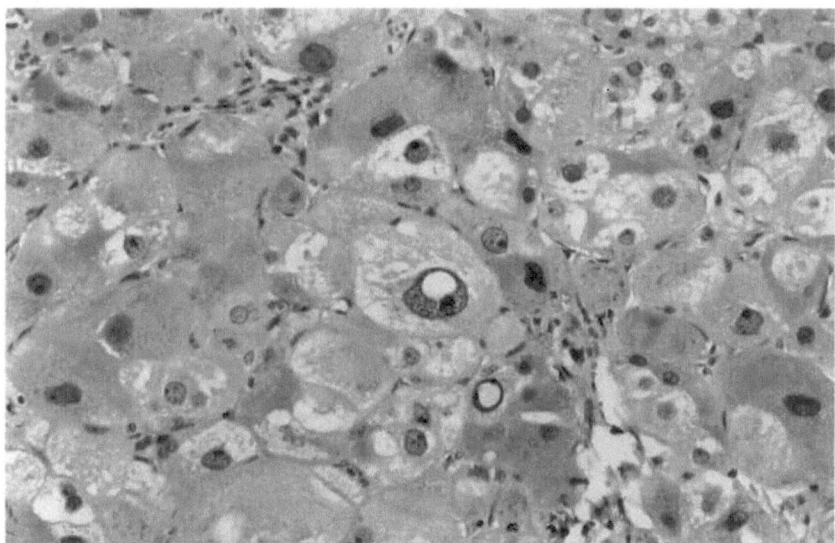

Fig. 29. Adrenal cortical adenoma with Cushing syndrome. Note moderate nuclear enlargement with occasional pseudoinclusions. Some tumour cells also contain faint granular brown pigment consistent with lipofuscin

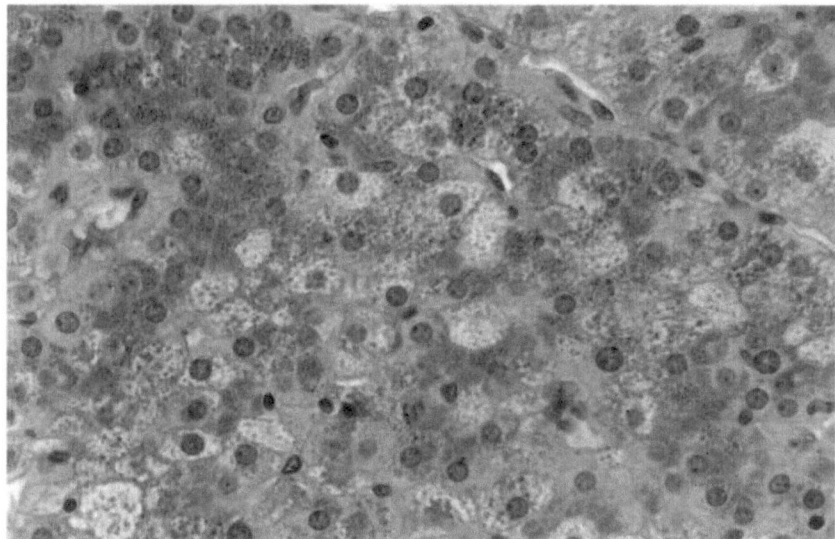

Fig. 30. Pigmented ("black") adenoma of adrenal gland associated with Cushing syndrome. Macroscopically, the tumour was jet-black on cross section. Cells contain abundant granular brown pigment representing lipofuscin

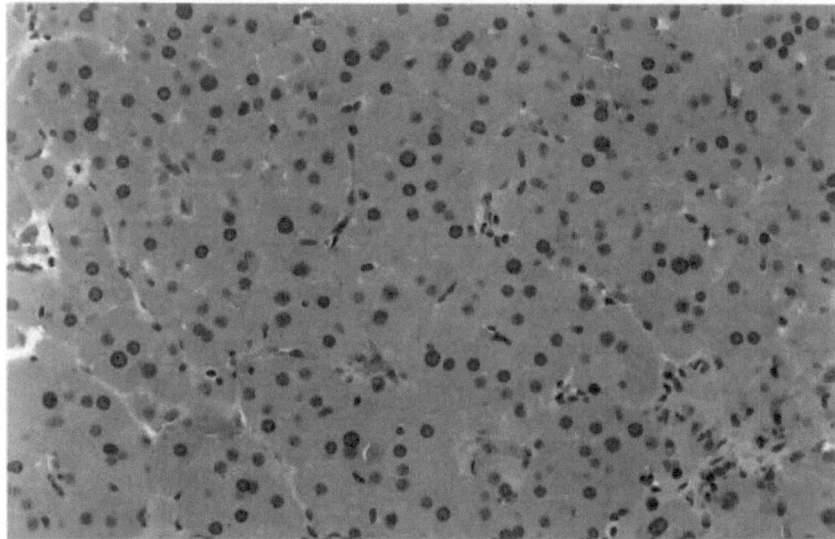

Fig. 31. Oncocytic adrenal cortical adenoma. Tumour cells have abundant granular pink cytoplasm. Tumour was mahogany-brown on cross section. There was no endocrinological evidence of hyperfunction

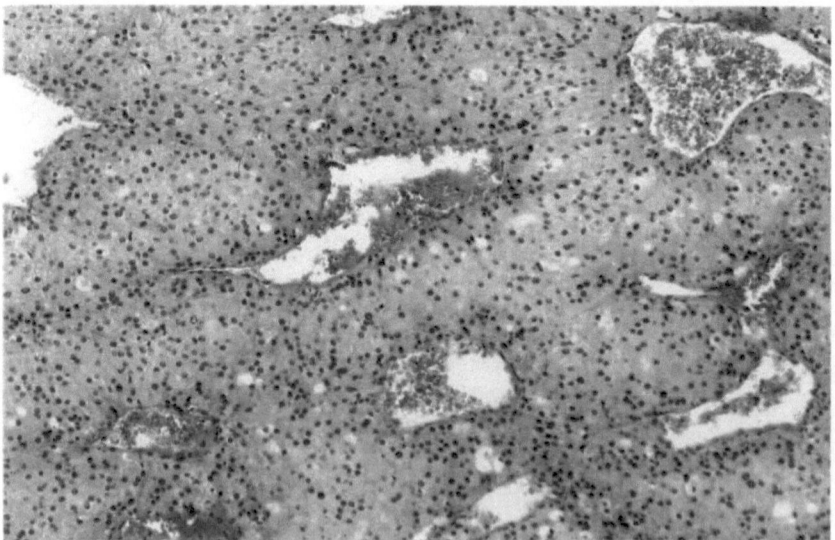

Fig. 32. Adrenal cortical carcinoma. Broad, anastomosing trabeculae with delicate sinusoidal lining. Lack of significant nuclear pleomorphism

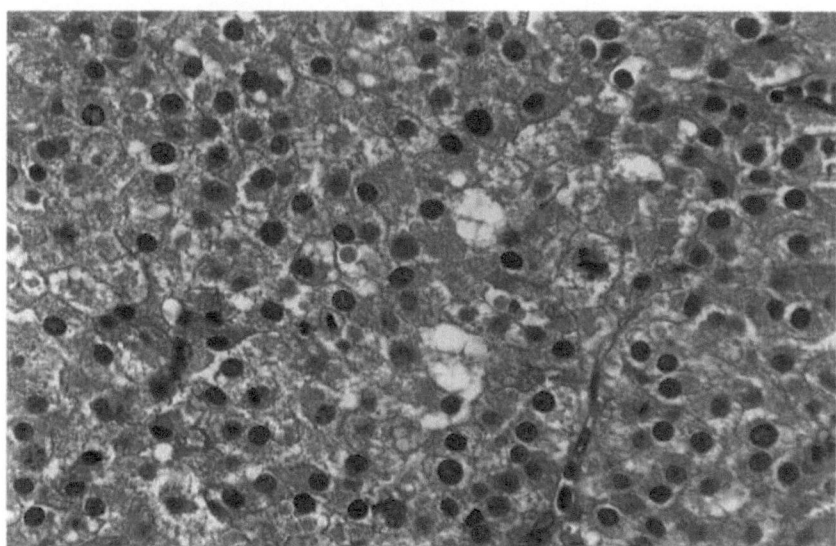

Fig. 33. Adrenal cortical carcinoma. A more diffuse or solid growth pattern with cells having compact, eosinophilic cytoplasm. Mitotic figure

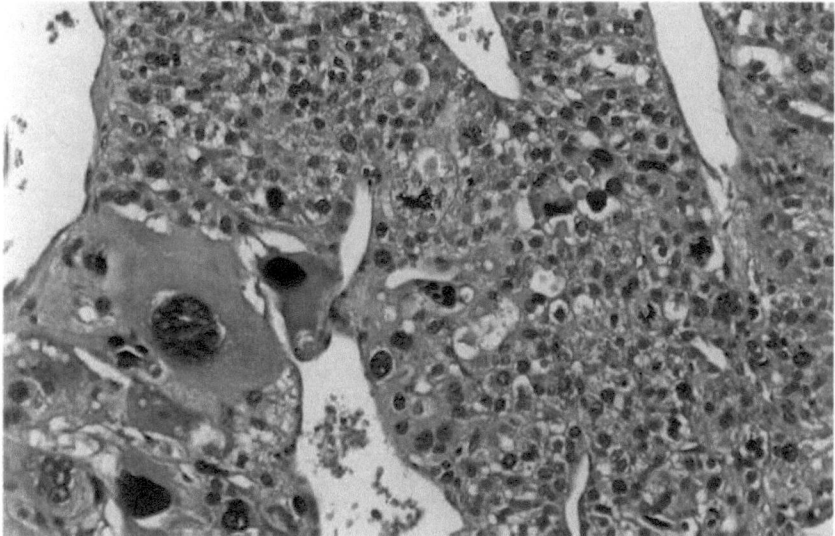

Fig. 34. Adrenal cortical carcinoma. Marked nuclear pleomorphism and numerous mitotic figures. Tumour also had few intracytoplasmic hyaline globules

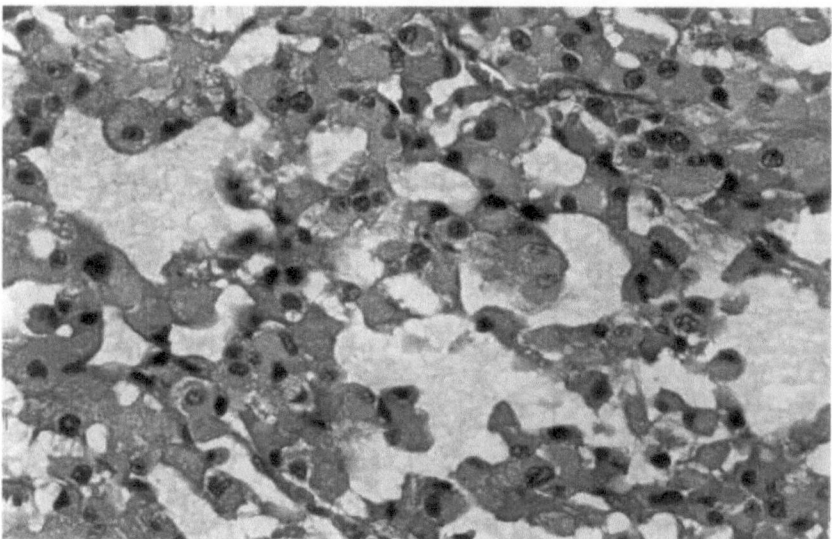

Fig. 35. Adrenal cortical carcinoma. Areas with myxoid pattern

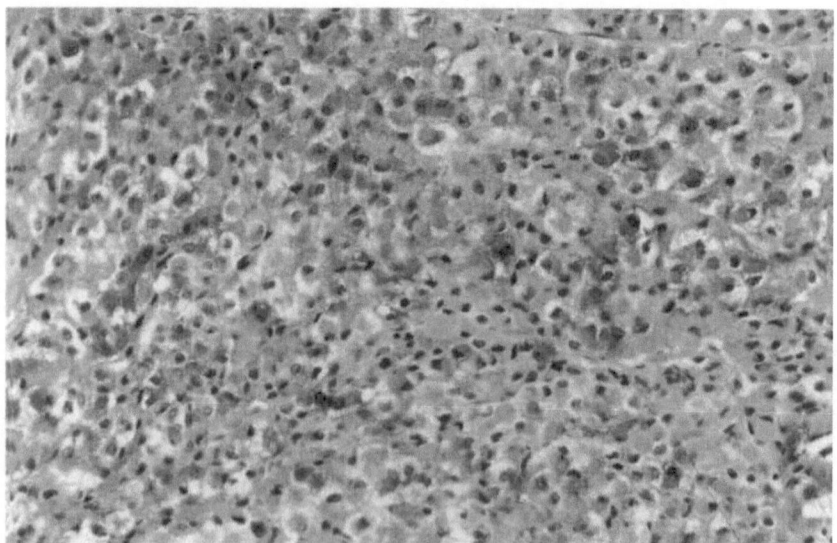

Fig. 36. Adrenal cortical carcinoma. Positive immunostaining for synaptophysin. The tumour was mistakenly classified as a pheochromocytoma

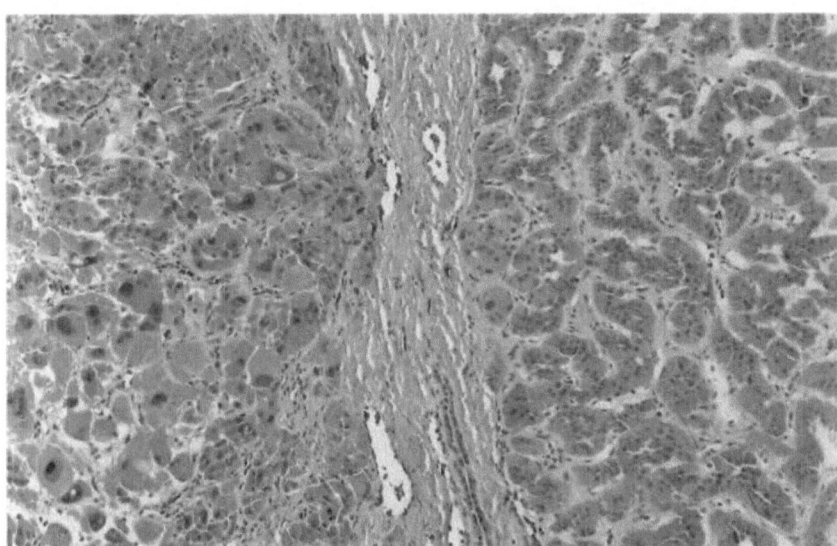

Fig. 37. Adrenal cortical nodule or adenoma. Clinically nonfunctional. The gland had multiple smaller cortical nodules, here with two in juxtaposition

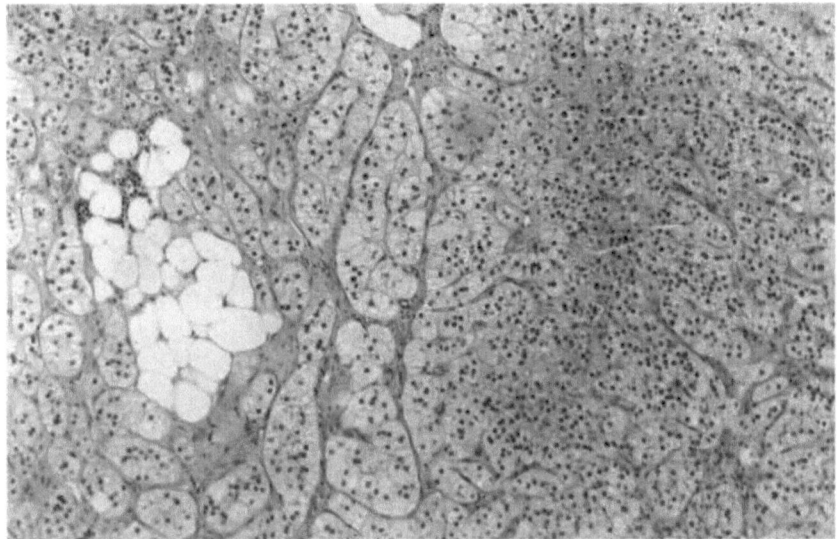

Fig. 38. Adrenal cortical nodule or adenoma. Incidentally discovered and clinically nonfunctional. Small focus of myelolipomatous metaplasia

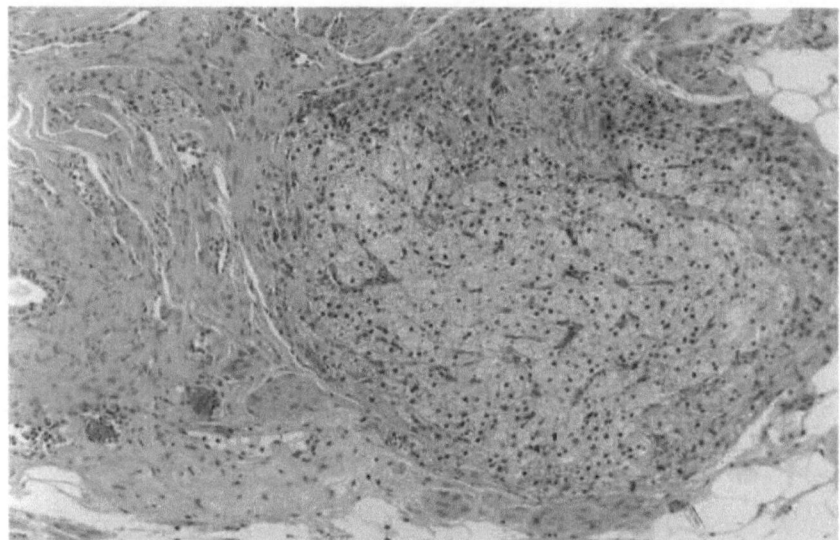

Fig. 39. Heterotopic adrenal cortex nodule near hilum of ovary

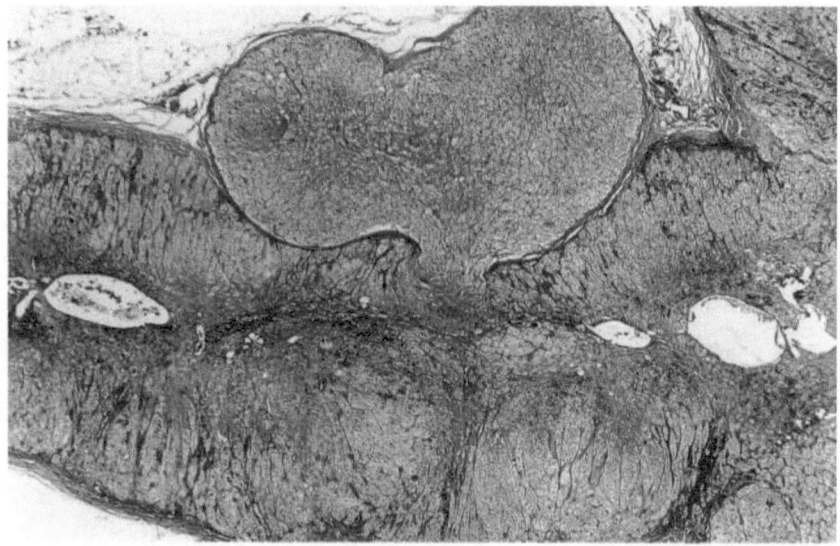

Fig. 40. Nodular adrenal gland. From a patient with multiple endocrine neoplasia syndrome type 1 (MEN1). Cortical extrusion has a mushroom configuration

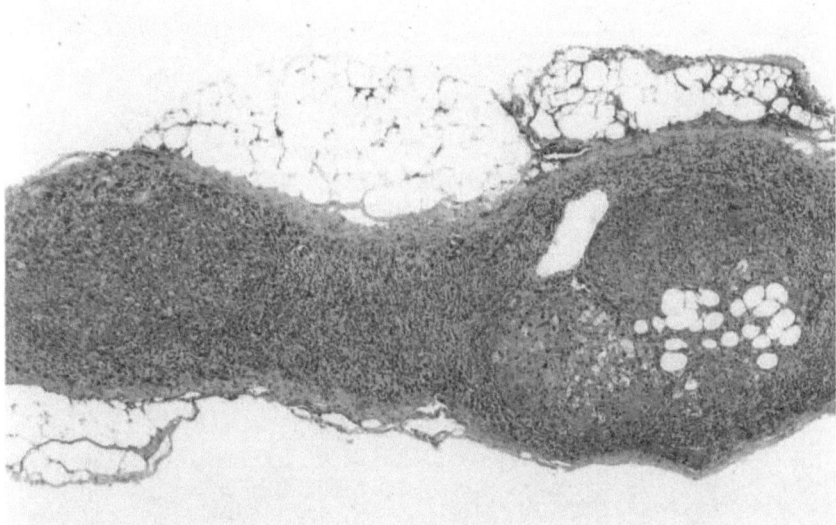

Fig. 41. Primary pigmented nodular adrenocortical disease (PPNAD). A rare primary form of hypercortisolism. Macroscopically, there were numerous, small, brown to black nodules studding the cortex. Internodular cortex is atrophic. Lipomatous component in nodule on right

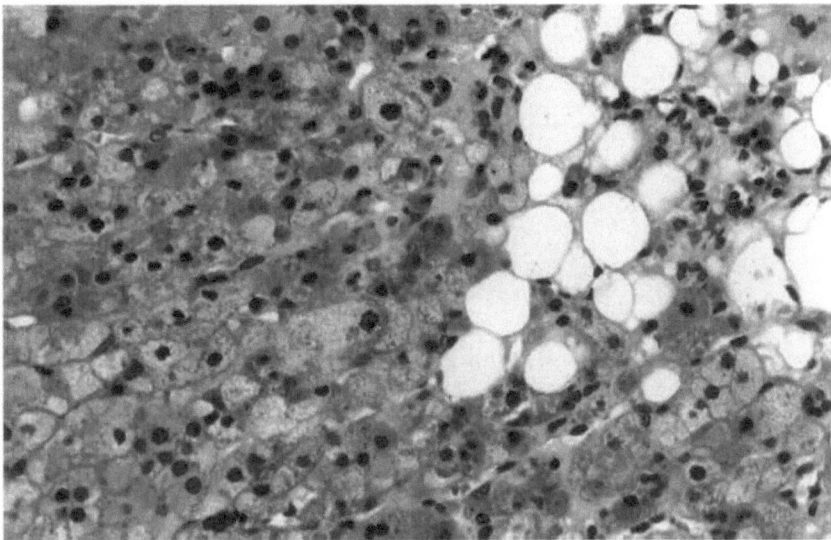

Fig. 42. Primary pigmented nodular adrenocortical disease (PPNAD). Most nodules are composed of cells with compact eosinophilic cytoplasm and variable amounts of granular brown pigment consistent with lipofuscin

100

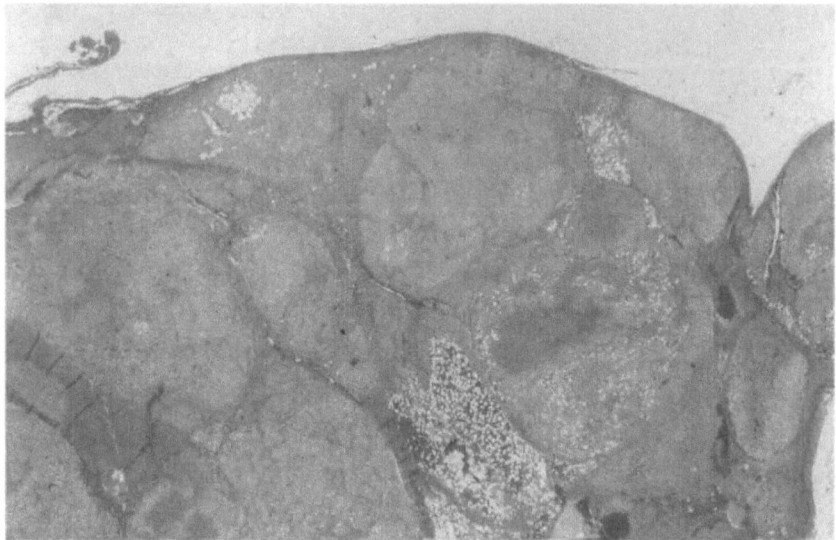

Fig. 43. Macronodular hyperplasia with marked adrenal enlargement (MHMAE). A rare cause of primary hypercortisolism. Both adrenal glands were markedly enlarged (combined weight 94 gms) with multiple cortical nodules of various size. Myelolipomatous metaplasia. Metaplastic bone was also present

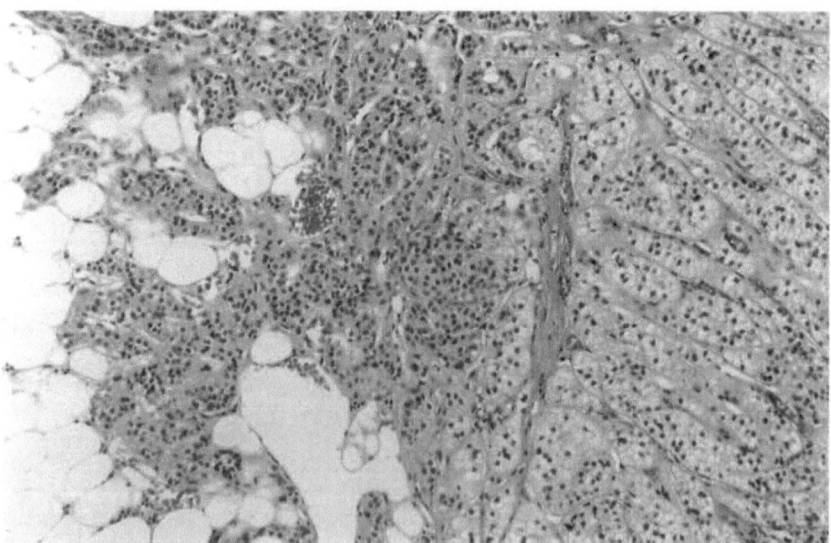

Fig. 44. Macronodular hyperplasia with marked adrenal enlargement (MHMAE). There were multiple hyperplastic cortical nodules with some extra-adrenal extension of cortical cells into periadrenal fat

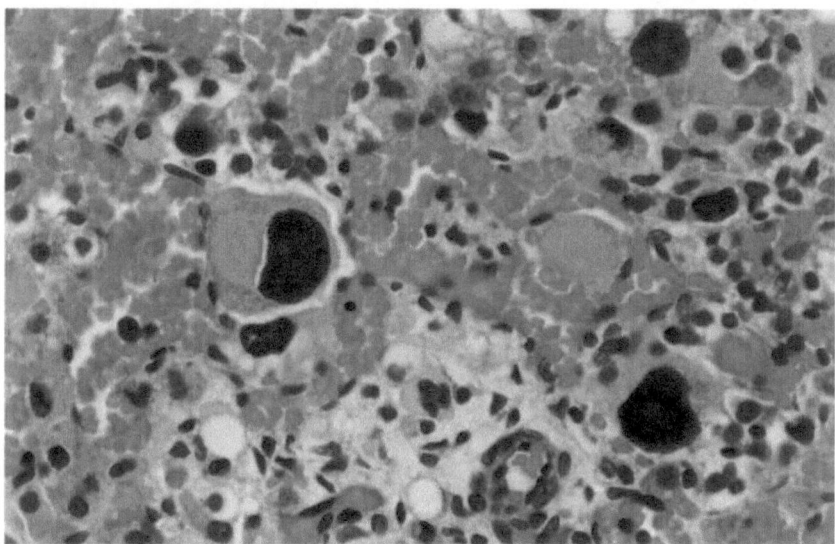

Fig. 45. Adrenal cytomegaly in Beckwith-Wiedemann syndrome. Some nuclei of foetal cortical cells in other areas also had pseudoinclusions

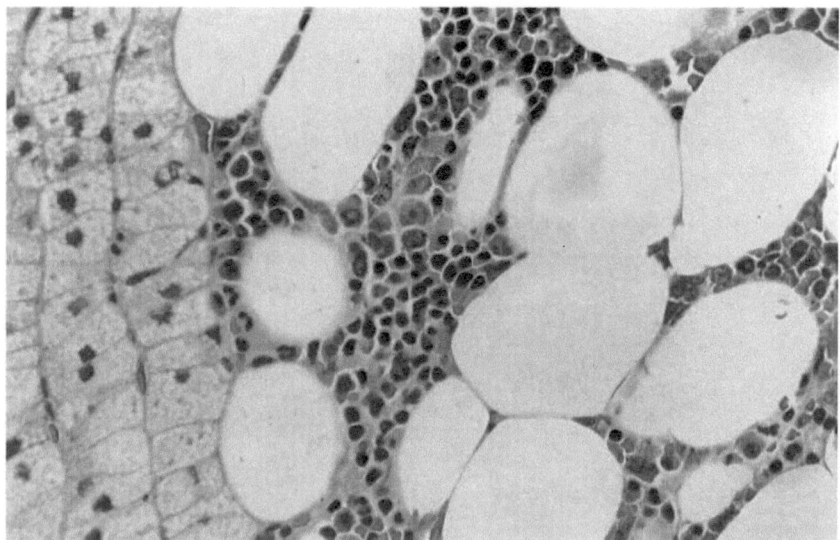

Fig. 46. Adrenal myelolipoma. Myeloid and erythroid cells are present along with mature adipose tissue. Megakaryocytes were present in other fields. Cortex is present on left side

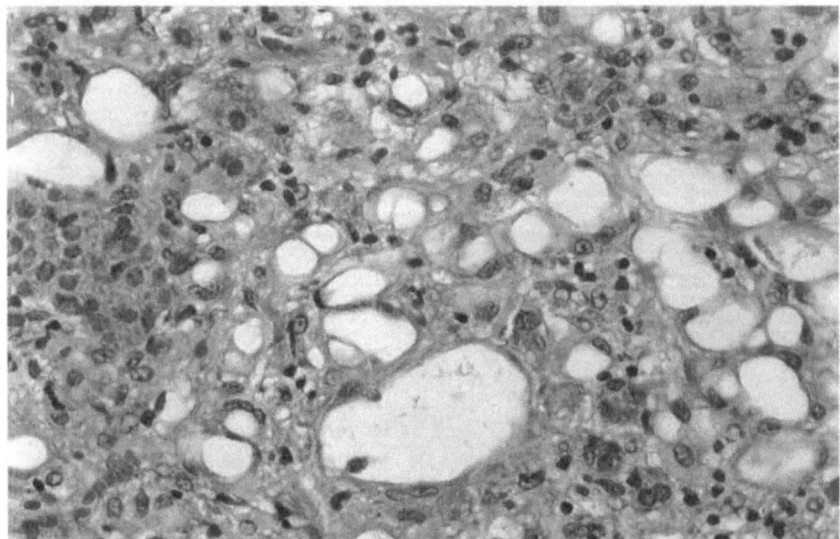

Fig. 47. Adenomatoid tumour of adrenal gland. Cytoplasmic vacuoles give a sieve-like or glandular appearance. Some cortical cells are entrapped

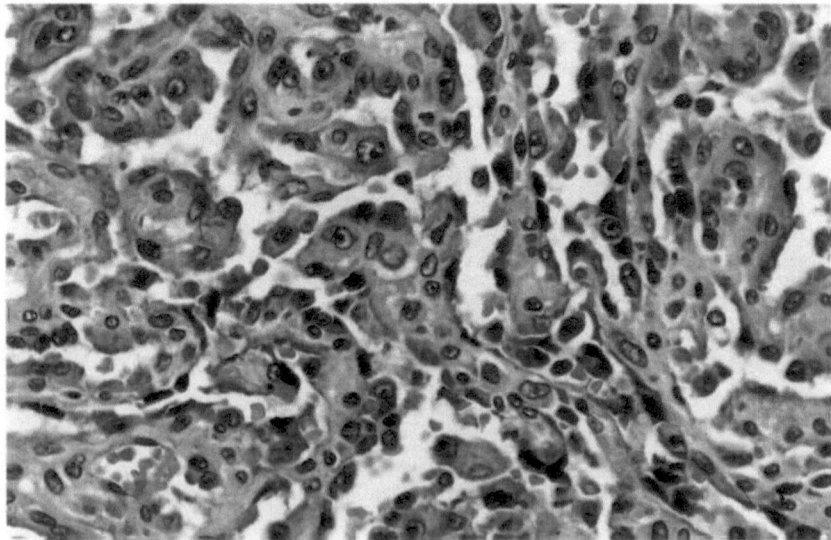

Fig. 48. Angiosarcoma of adrenal gland. Tumour is very vasoformative with papillary tufts lined by malignant endothelial cells

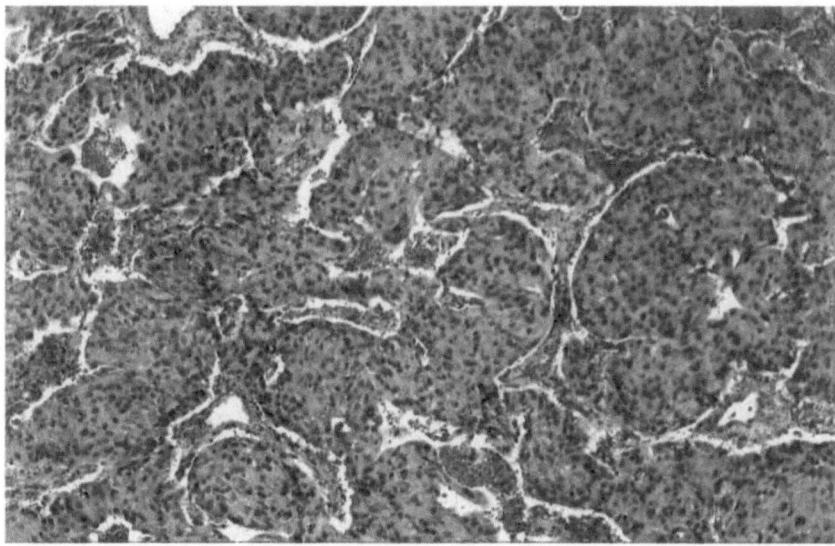

Fig. 49. Pheochromocytoma. Anastomosing trabecular pattern with prominent microvasculature

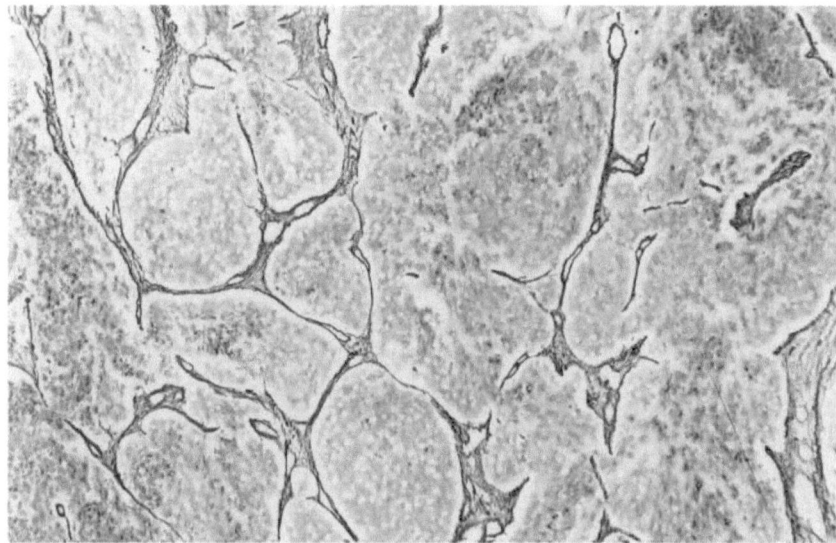

Fig. 50. Pheochromocytoma. Mixture of alveolar and anastomosing trabecular patterns is accentuated by stain for reticulum

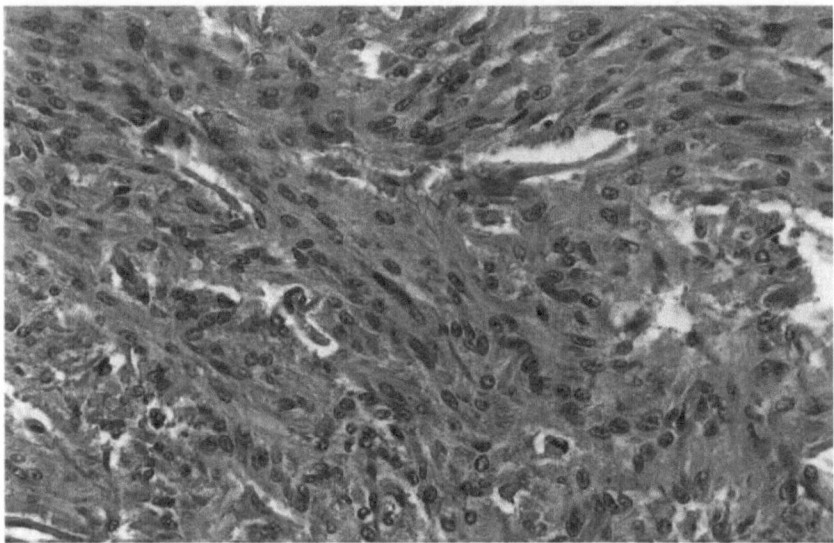

Fig. 51. Pheochromocytoma. Focally, this tumour has a spindle cell pattern with nuclei also being slightly elongate in the same axis

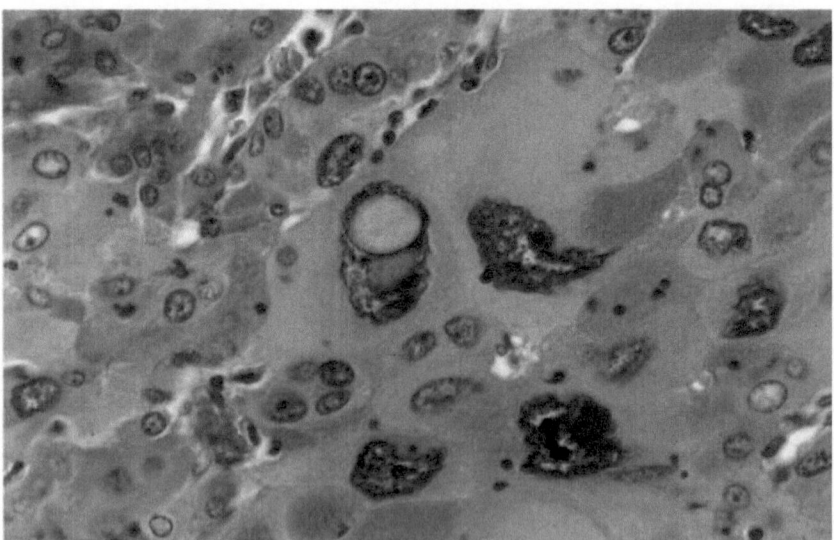

Fig. 52. Pheochromocytoma. Pleomorphic, hyperchromatic nuclei with one near centre of field having two nuclear pseudoinclusions

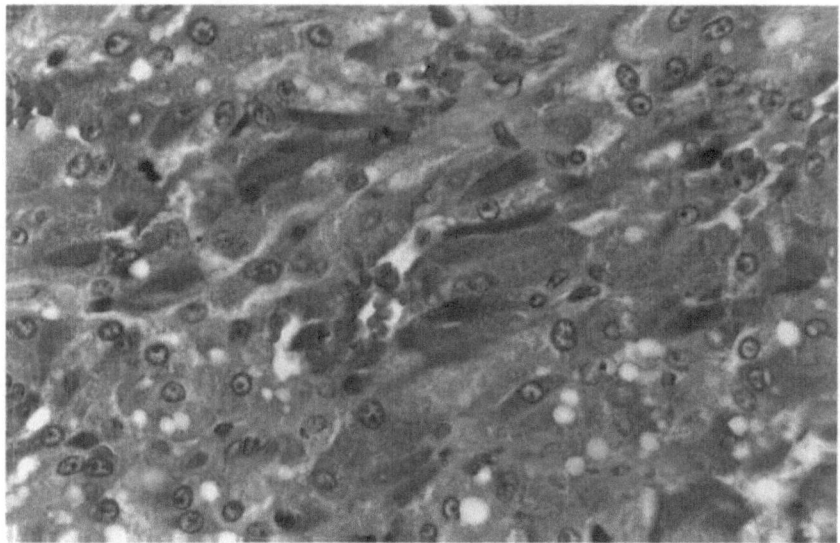

Fig. 53. Pheochromocytoma. Tumour cells have lavender cytoplasm with a myriad of pinpoint basophilic granules

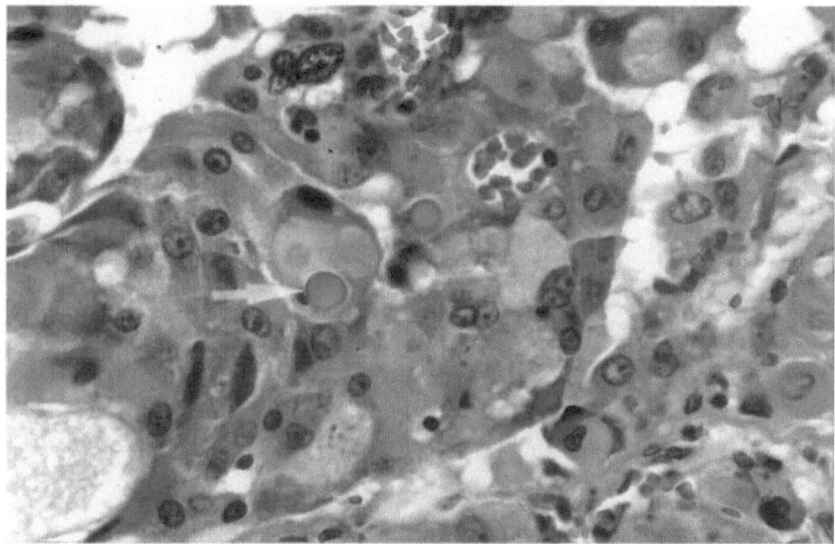

Fig. 54. Pheochromocytoma. Some tumour cells contain eosinophilic hyaline globules (*arrow*) which are PAS-positive and resistant to diastase predigestion

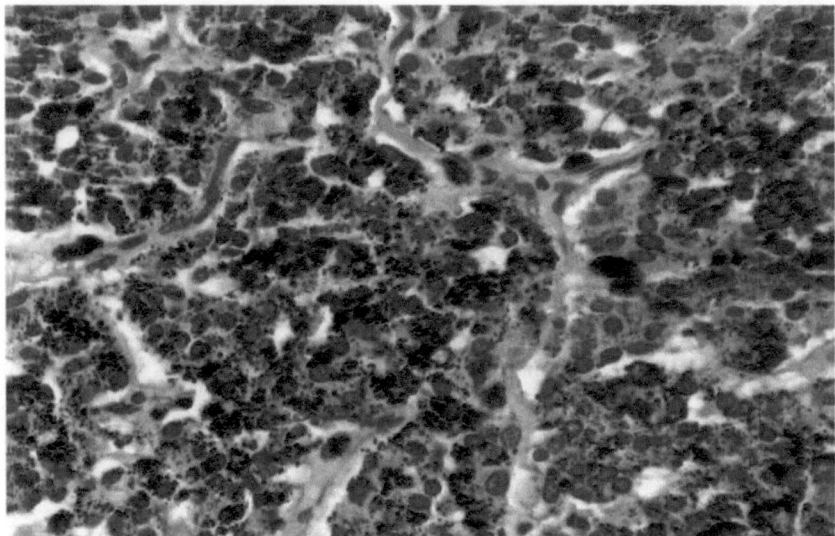

Fig. 55. Pigmented ("black") pheochromocytoma. Tumour cells contain abundant coarse granular pigment which proved to be neuromelanin. Tumour was jet-black and simulated a malignant melanoma

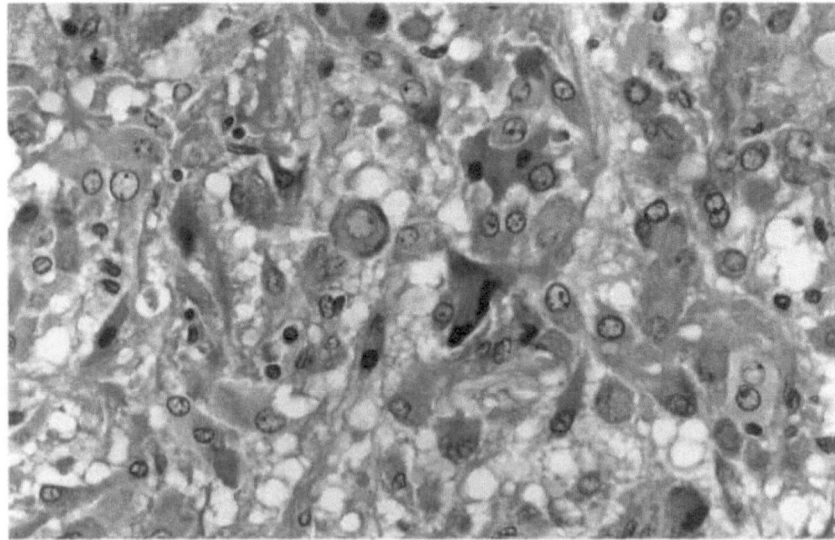

Fig. 56. Composite pheochromocytoma. Neuronal or ganglionic cells (*arrow*) are set within a fibrillar background. Basophilic material resembling Nissl substance. In other areas, tumour had typical histology for pheochromocytoma

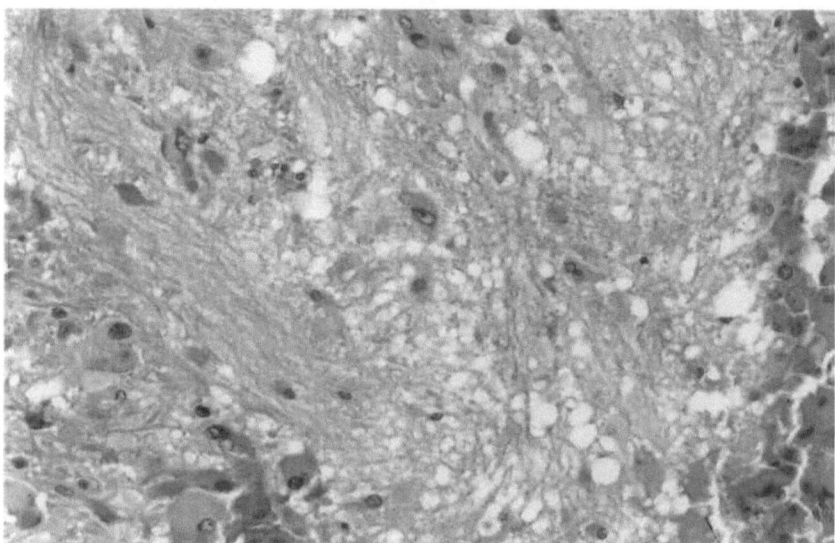

Fig. 57. Composite pheochromocytoma. Broad mats of fibrillary matrix resembling neuropil and few ganglion-like cells

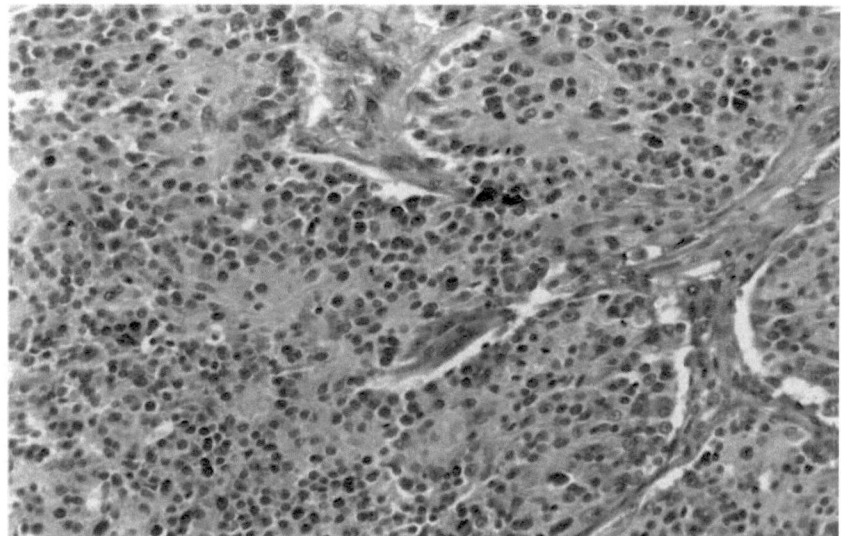

Fig. 58. Composite pheochromocytoma. Small, neuroblast-like cells are set within a scant fibrillar matrix. Some tumour cells have neuronal or ganglionic features

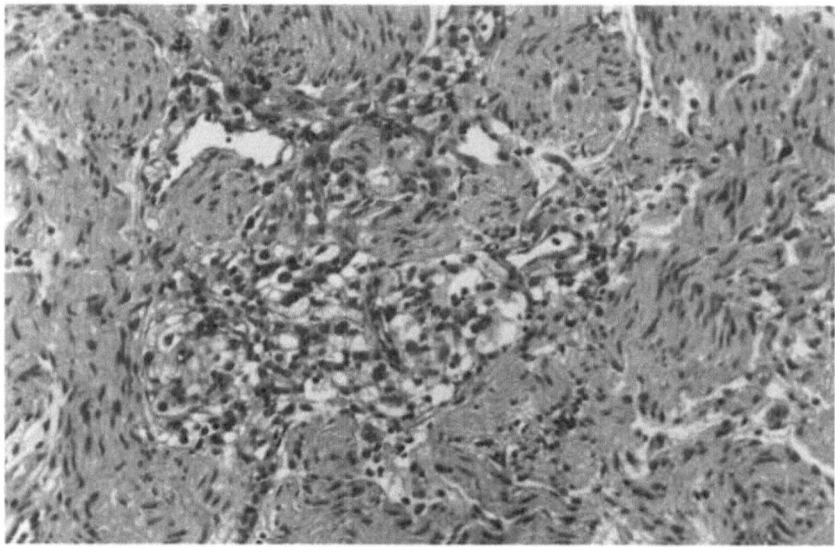

Fig. 59. Composite pheochromocytoma. Tumour is composed of pheochromocytoma and ganglioneuroma. Mature ganglion cells were present in other areas of tumour

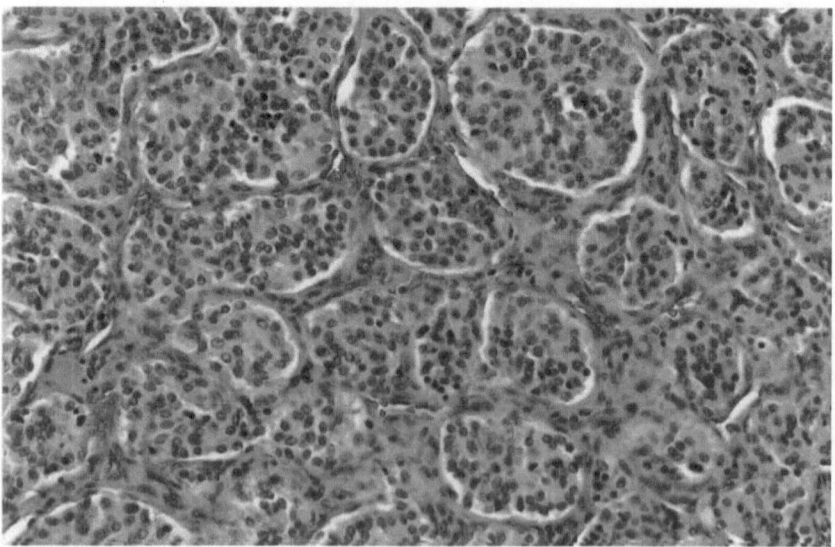

Fig. 60. Carotid body paraganglioma. Characteristic nesting or alveolar pattern with formation of "Zellballen" (cell clumps)

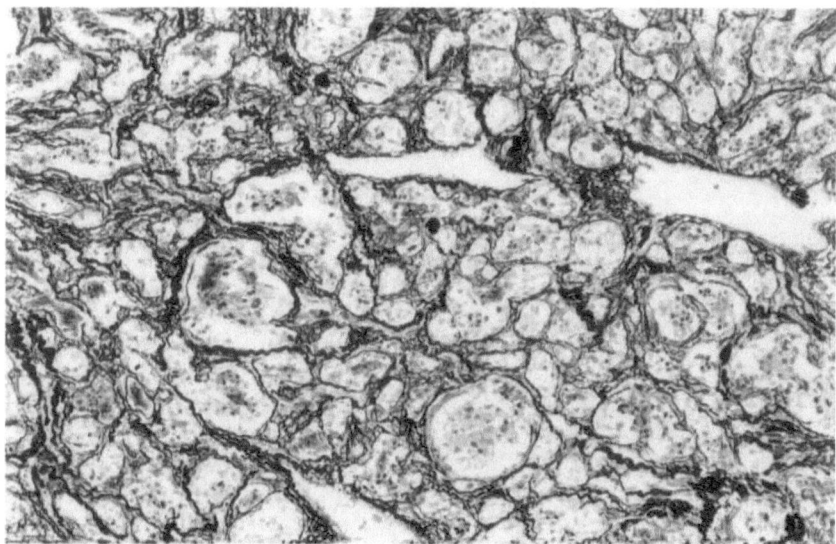

Fig. 61. Carotid body paraganglioma. Nesting or organoid pattern is accentuated by staining for reticulum

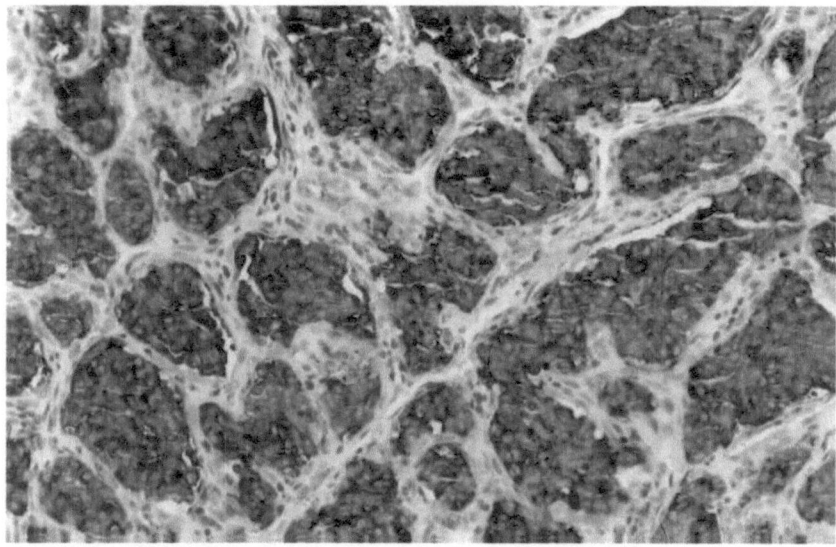

Fig. 62. Carotid body paraganglioma. Immunostain for chromogranin A is strongly positive within cytoplasm of neoplastic chief cells

110

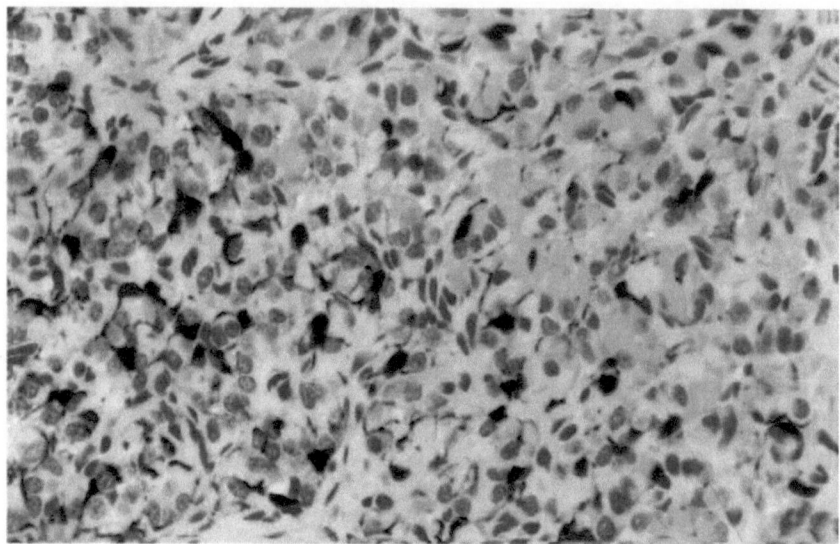

Fig. 63. Jugulotympanic paraganglioma. Plump spindle to dendritic sustentacular cells show positive nuclear and cytoplasmic staining for S-100 protein

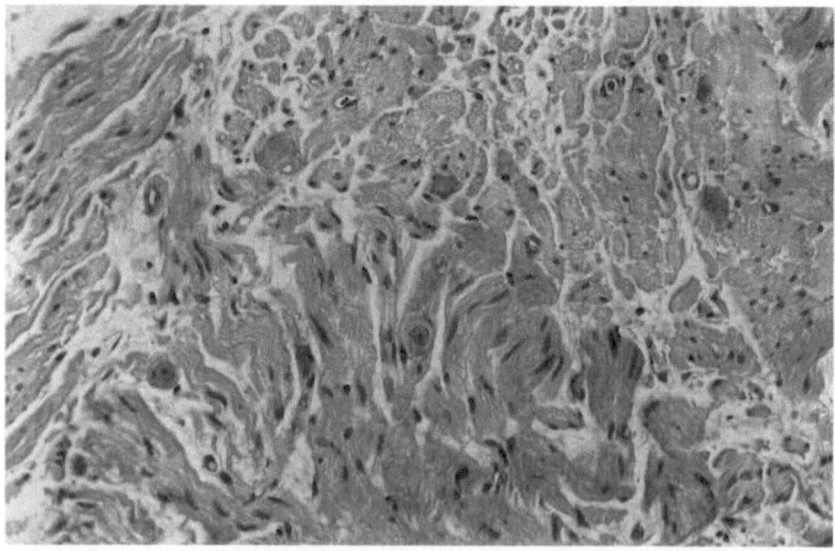

Fig. 64. Ganglioneuroma. Fascicular arrangement of Schwann cells and few ganglion cells in this field

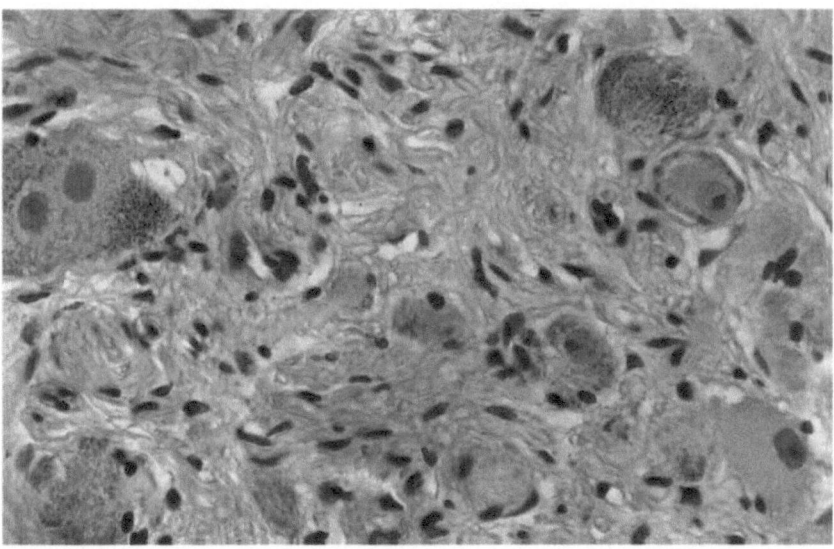

Fig. 65. Ganglioneuroma. Some ganglion cells in this field contain finely granular brown pigment consistent with lipofuscin or neuromelanin. Occasional cell has prominent Nissl substance

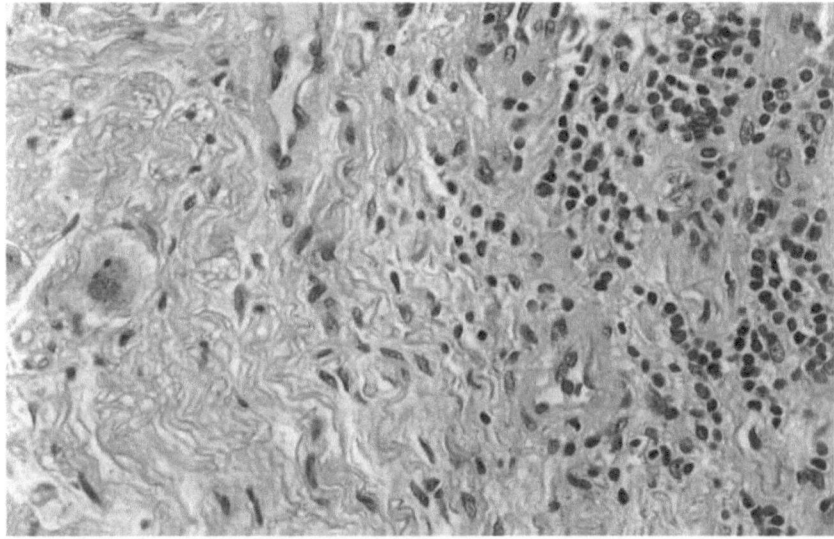

Fig. 66. Ganglioneuroma. Perivascular infiltrate by lymphocytes on right side should not be mistaken for neuroblasts

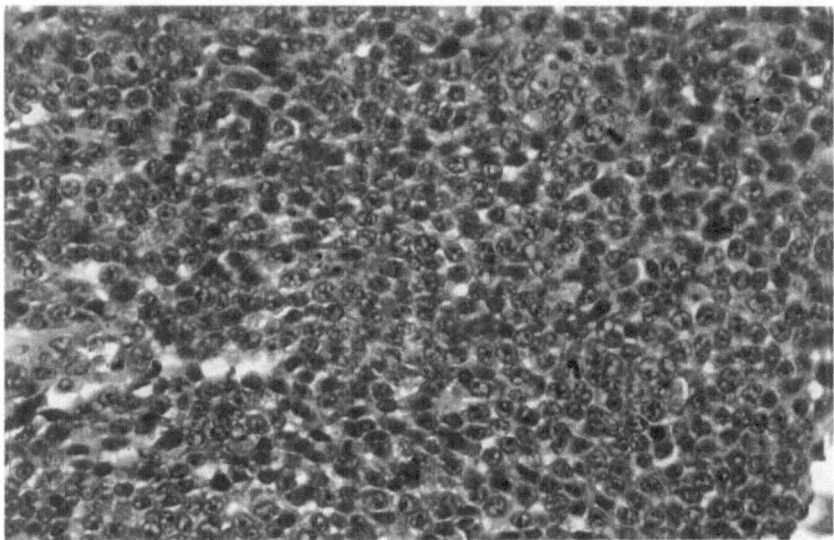

Fig. 67. Neuroblastoma. Tumour had diffuse sheets of primitive neuroblasts with high mitotic rate. Tumour was stroma-poor with unfavourable prognosis using the Shimada age-linked classification

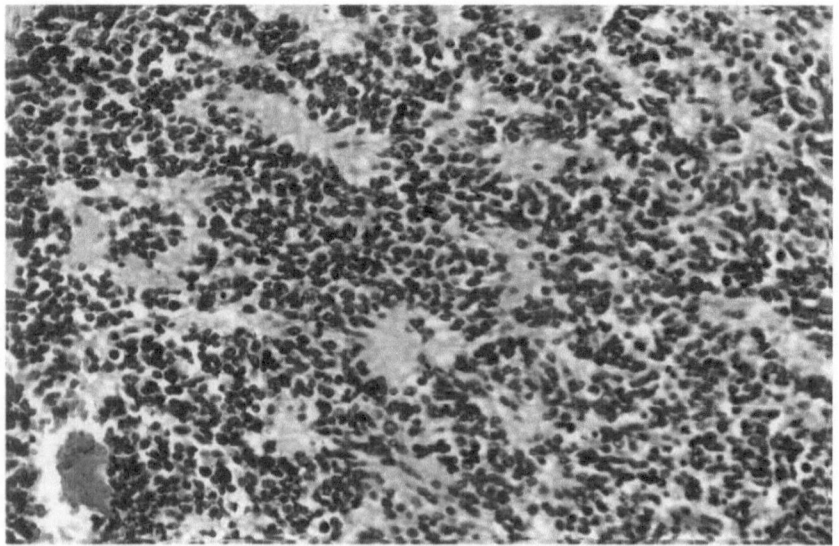

Fig. 68. Neuroblastoma. Tumour has numerous Homer Wright rosettes

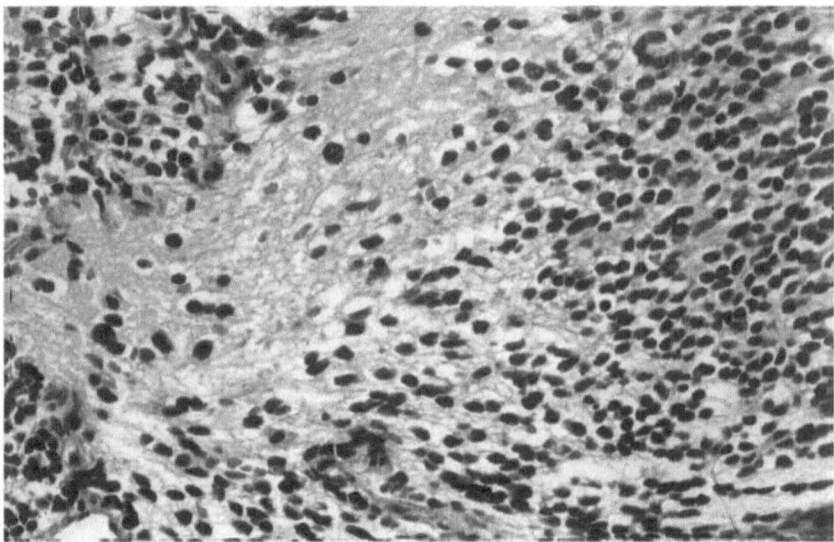

Fig. 69. Neuroblastoma. Tumour has relatively abundant fibrillary matrix resembling neuropil and is undifferentiated, in terms of showing no maturation into ganglion cells

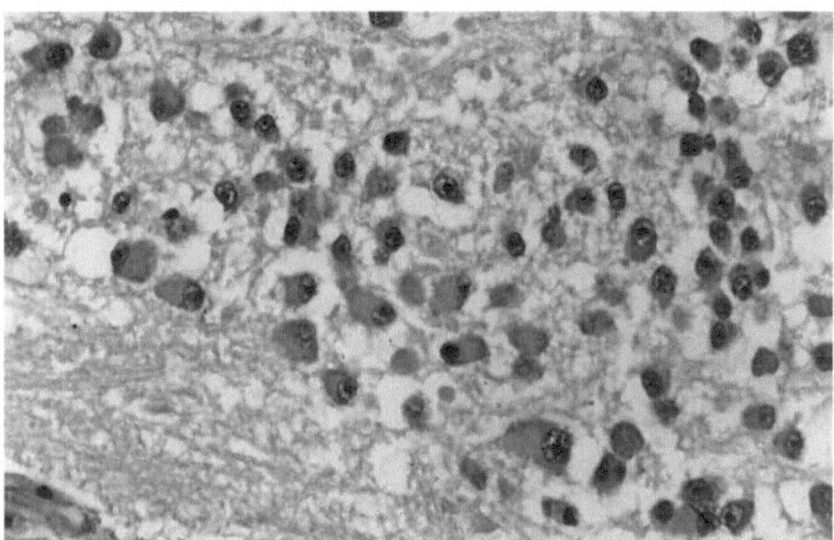

Fig. 70. Ganglioneuroblastoma. Immature ganglion cells are set within a rich fibrillary background resembling neuropil. Tumour was stroma-poor with favourable prognosis

114

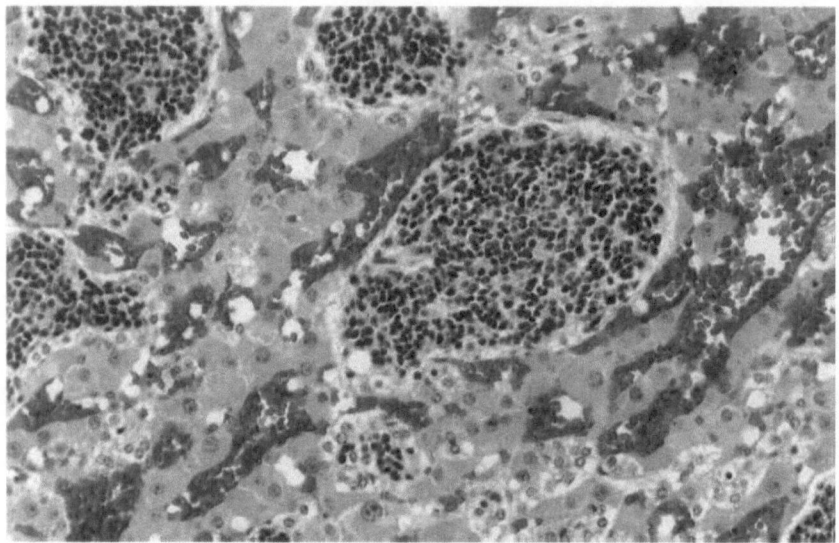

Fig. 71. Neuroblastic nodules in foetal adrenal gland. These are part of normal developmental anatomy. Some cells showed maturation into small nests of pale-staining chromaffin cells

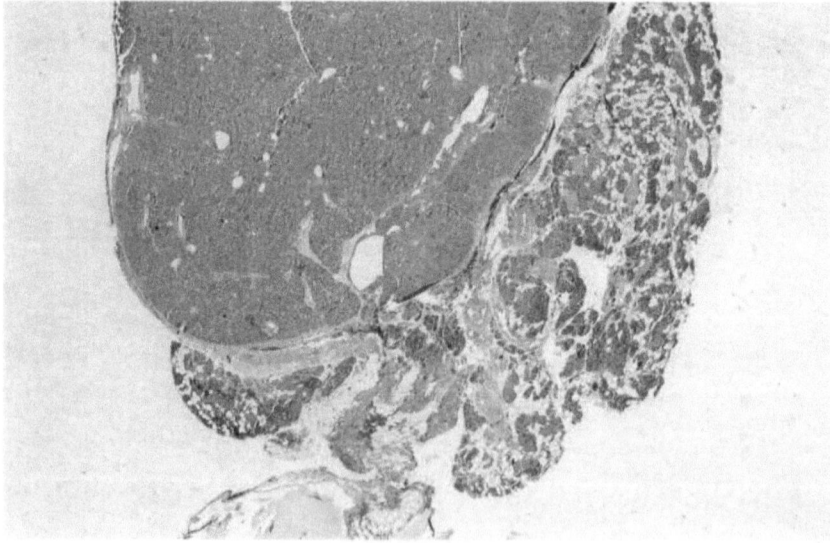

Fig. 72. Chief cell adenoma. A rim of normocellular parathyroid tissue is present adjacent to this relatively small chief cell adenoma

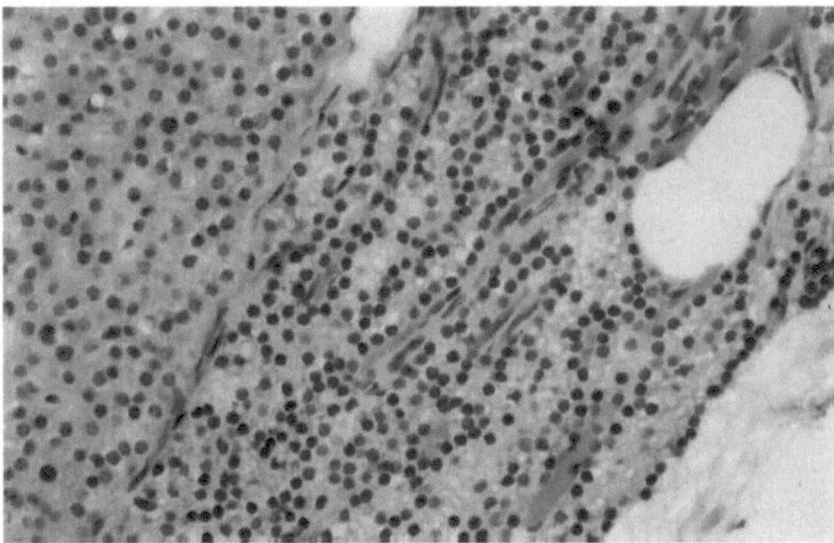

Fig. 73. Chief cell adenoma. The adenoma is separated from the adjacent normal parathyroid by a thin, fibrous capsule. In contrast to the adenoma cells, which have a faintly eosinophilic cytoplasm, the normal chief cells have a clear appearance due to the presence of large, lipid-containing vacuoles

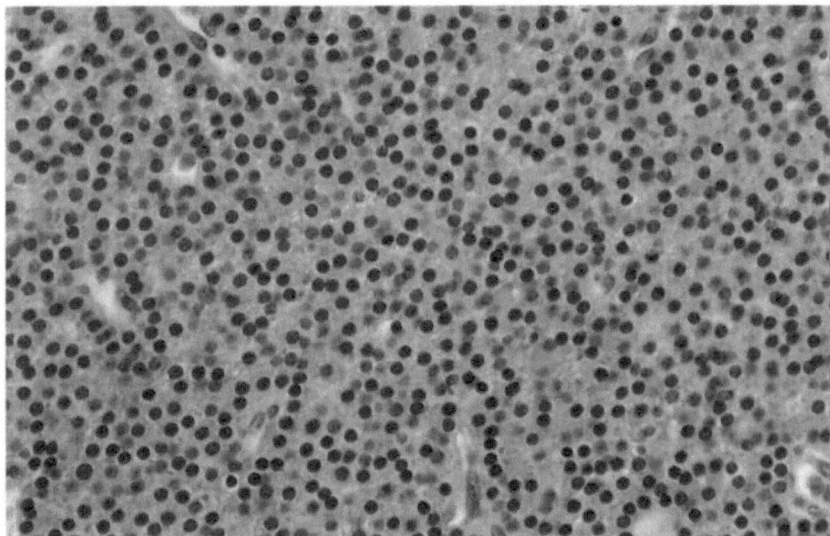

Fig. 74. Chief cell adenoma. The tumour cells have a faintly eosinophilic cytoplasm with round nuclei and dense chromatin

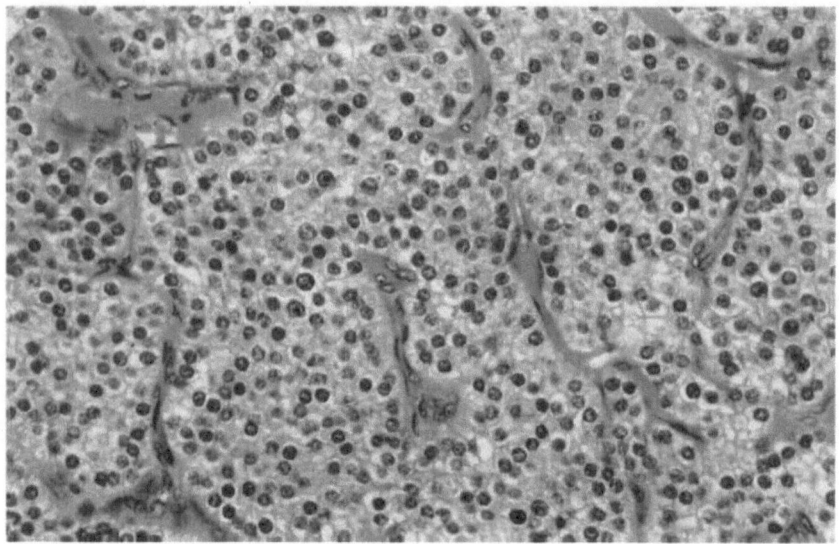

Fig. 75. Chief cell adenoma. The tumour cells have a somewhat clear appearance but lack the multiple cytoplasmic vacuoles seen in cases of clear cell adenoma

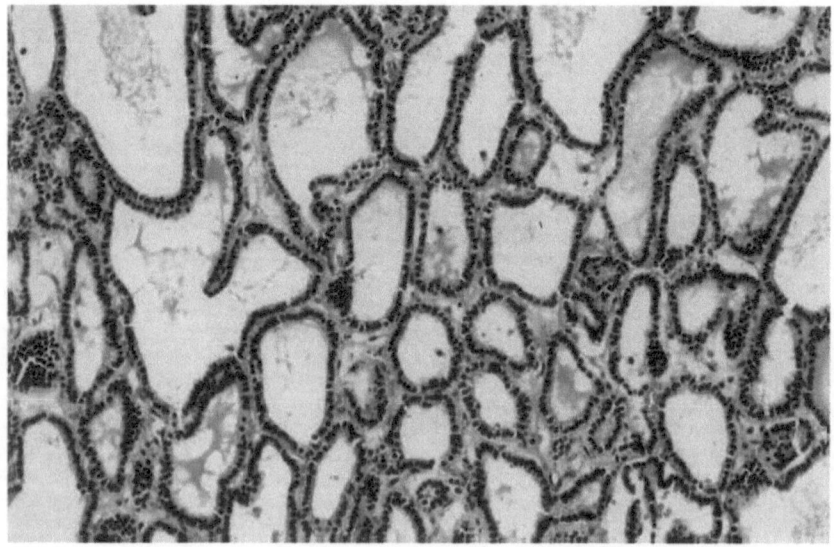

Fig. 76. Chief cell adenoma. The tumour cells are arranged in a follicular pattern throughout. Most of the follicles have an "empty" appearance

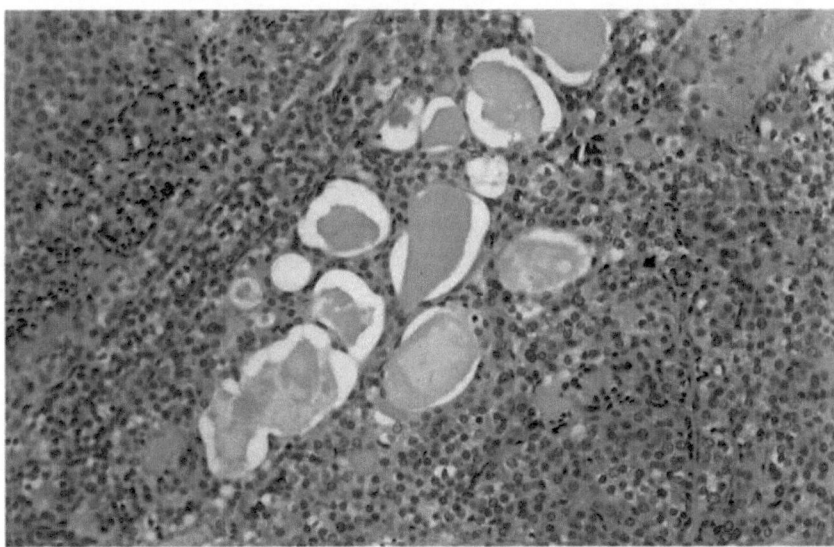

Fig. 77. Chief cell adenoma. The tumour cells in this case are present focally in a follicular pattern. Many of the follicles contain an eosinophilic colloid-like material

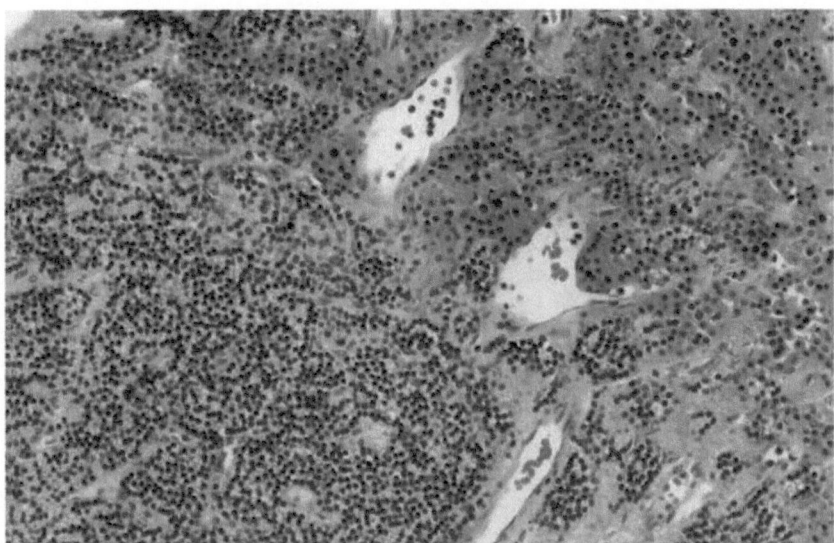

Fig. 78. Chief cell adenoma. This tumour is composed predominantly of chief cells
with scattered groups of oncocytes. The latter cells are characterised by the presence
of granular eosinophilic cytoplasm

118

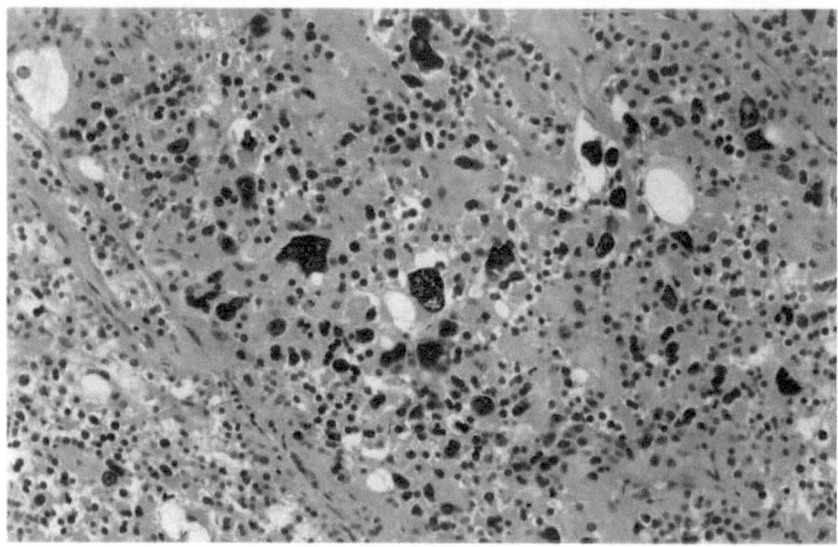

Fig. 79. Chief cell adenoma. This tumour has scattered cells with enlarged and irregularly shaped hyperchromatic nuclei

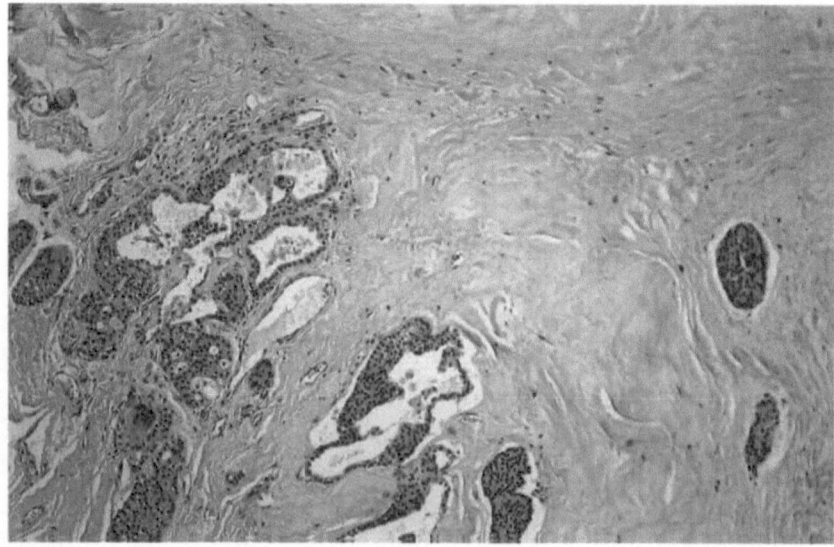

Fig. 80. Chief cell adenoma. The capsule of this degenerated adenoma is markedly thickened and contains groups of entrapped chief cells

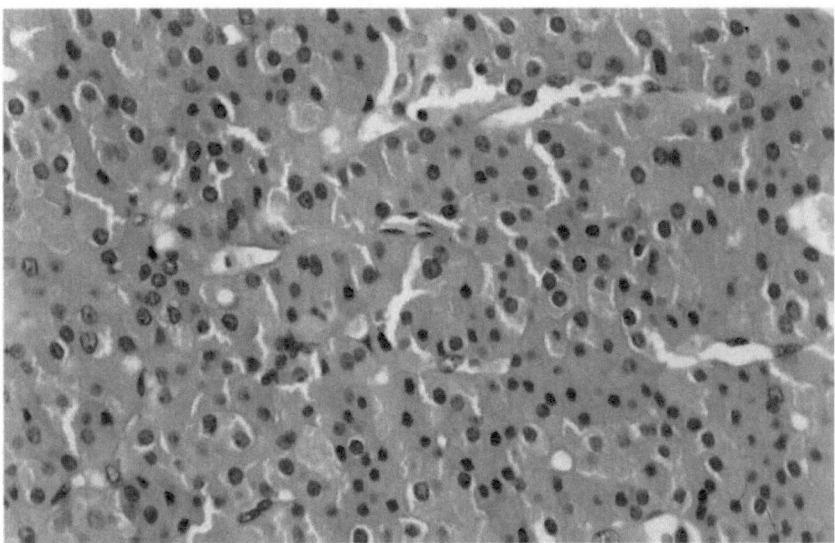

Fig. 81. Oncocytic adenoma. This tumour is composed exclusively of large cells with granular eosinophilic cytoplasm

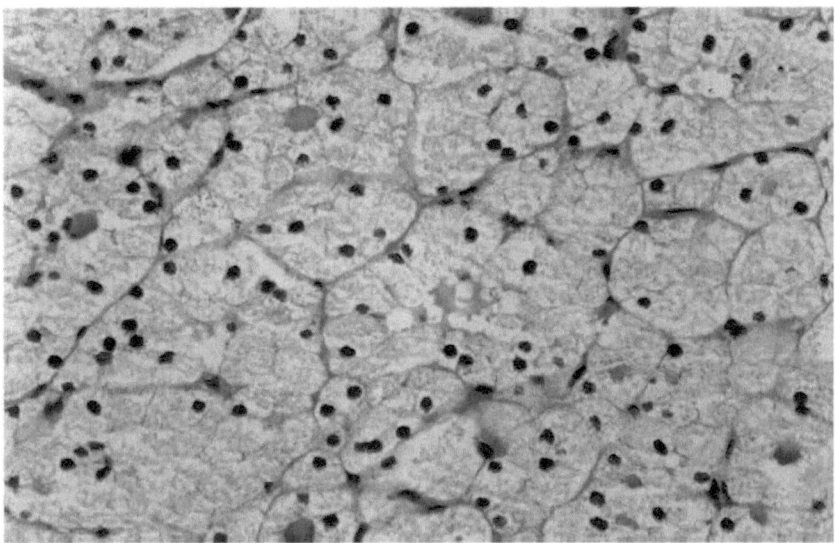

Fig. 82. Clear cell adenoma. This clear appearance of the tumour cells is due to the presence of multiple small cytoplasmic vacuoles

120

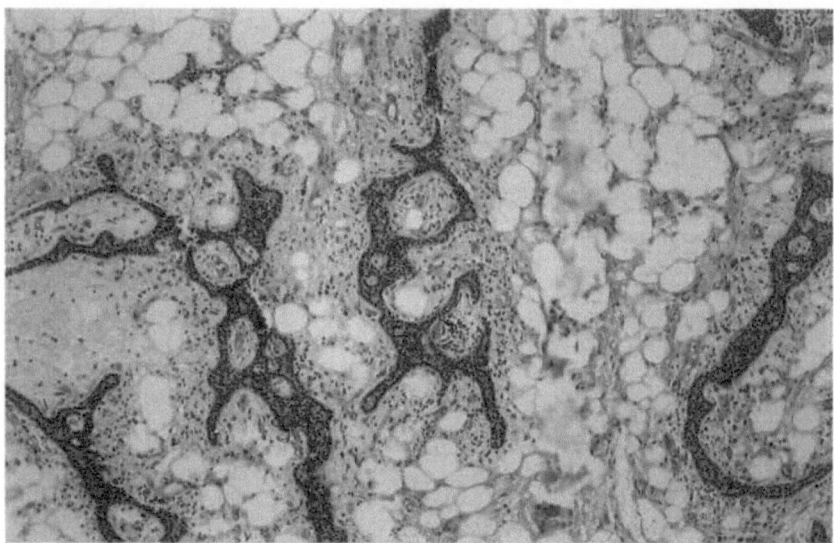

Fig. 83. Lipoadenoma. The chief cells are arranged in thin, branching, cord-like arrangements. The stroma includes fat and fibrous tissue with areas of myxoid change

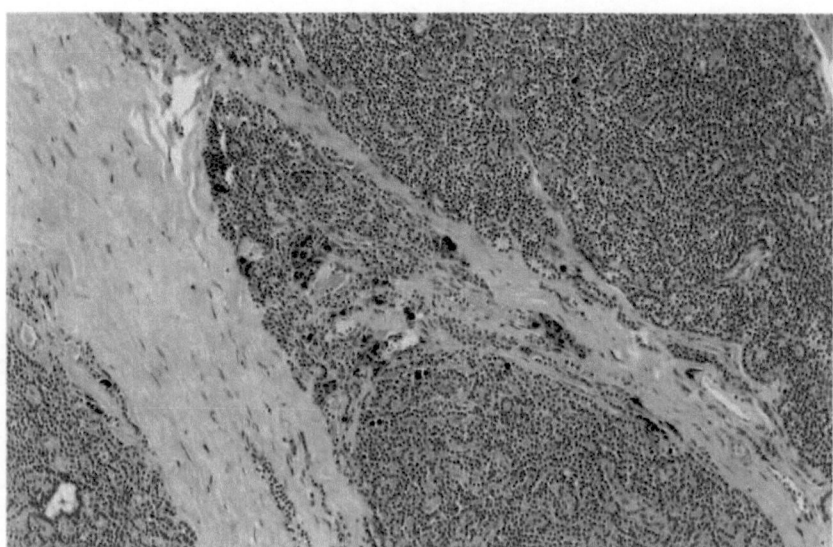

Fig. 84. Atypical adenoma. This chief cell adenoma is transected by broad bands of dense fibrous corrective tissue with areas of haemosiderin deposition. The tumour did not invade the adjacent normal tissues

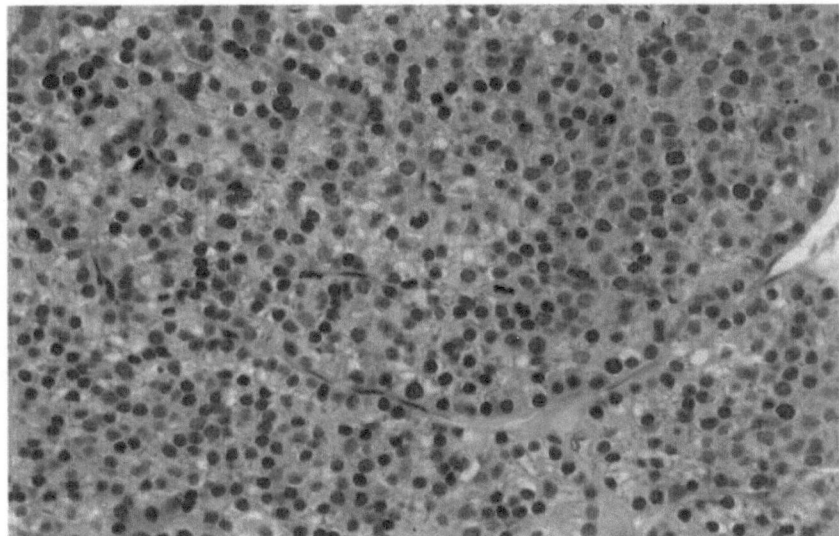

Fig. 85. Parathyroid carcinoma. This tumour is composed of a relatively monotonous population of chief cells with prominent mitotic activity. This tumour invaded the soft tissue of the neck

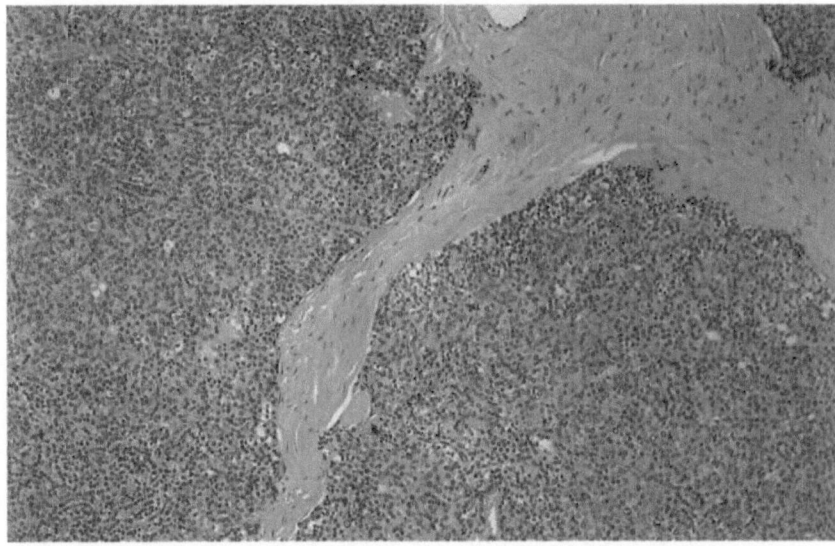

Fig. 86. Parathyroid carcinoma. This tumour is transected by broad bands of fibrous connective tissue. There was focal invasion of the soft tissues of the neck

122

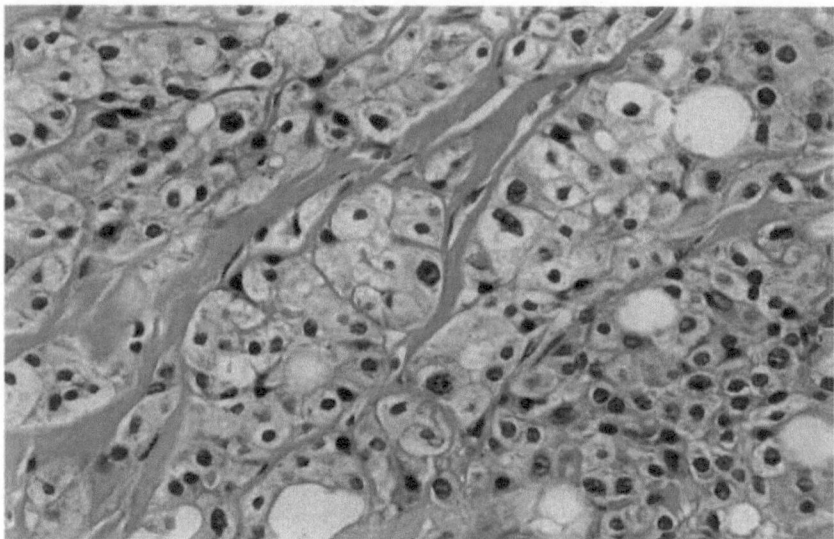

Fig. 87. Parathyroid carcinoma. This tumour is composed of groups of chief cells with pleomorphic nuclei. The cell groups are separated by relatively thin fibrous bands

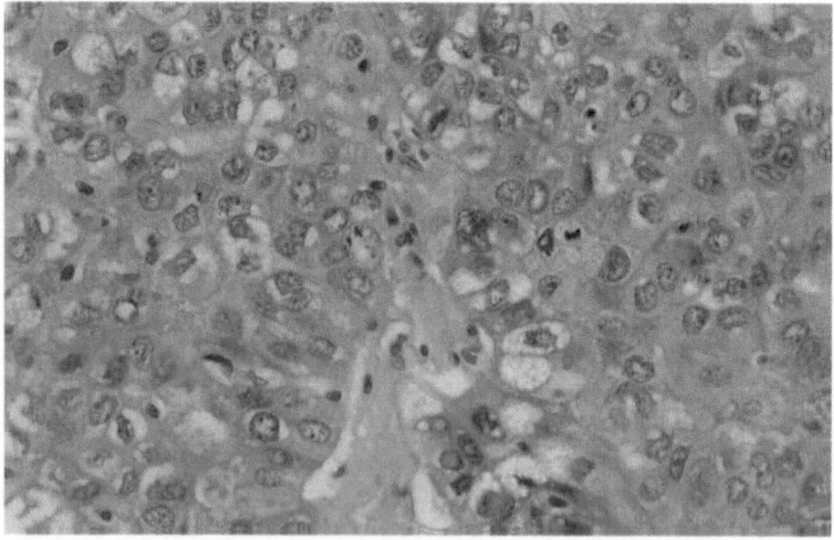

Fig. 88. Parathyroid carcinoma. This tumour is composed of pleomorphic chief cells with prominent mitotic activity

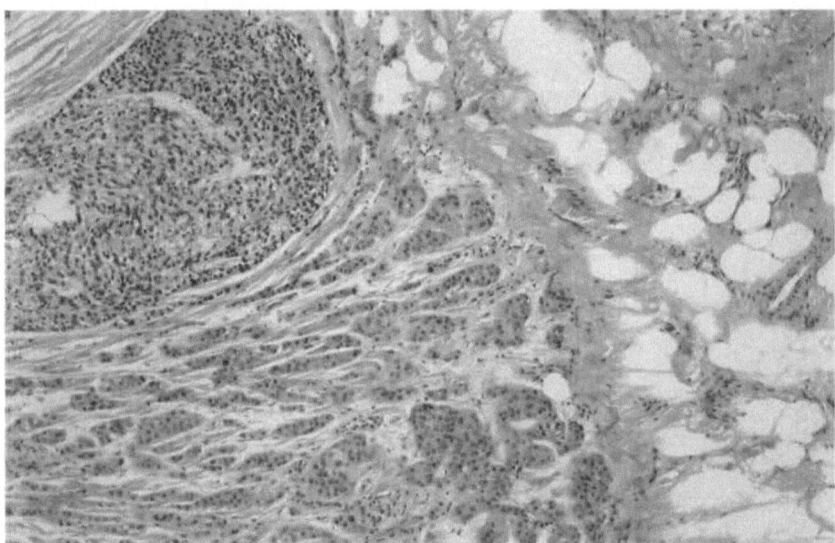

Fig. 89. Parathyroid carcinoma. This tumour infiltrates the adjacent adipose tissue

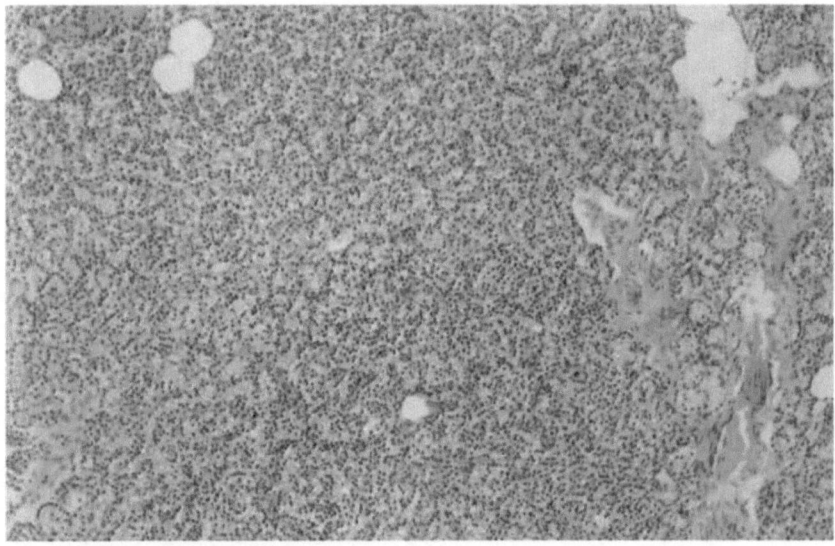

Fig. 90. Primary chief cell hyperplasia. The hyperplasia in this case has an exclusively diffuse growth pattern. The individual chief cells have a clear appearance

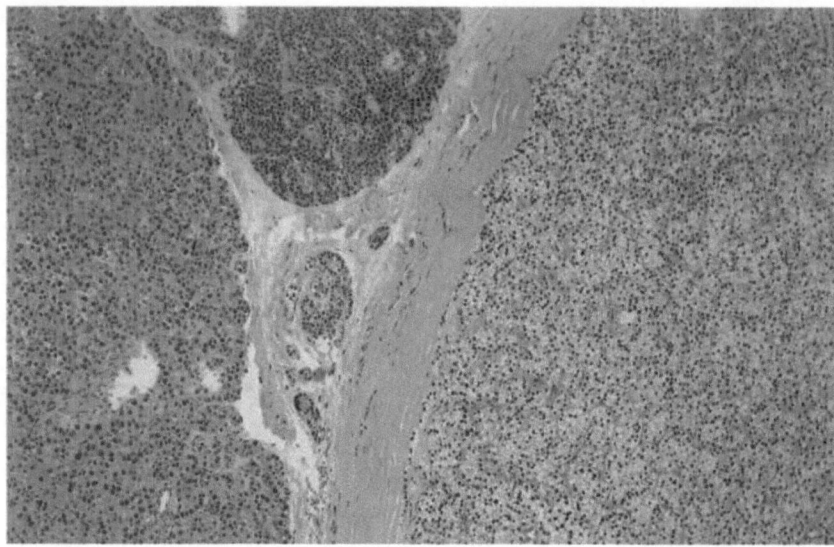

Fig. 91. Primary chief cell hyperplasia. The hyperplasia in this case is nodular. A single nodule composed of chief cells is separated from the adjacent diffusely hyperplastic chief cells by a thick fibrous capsule

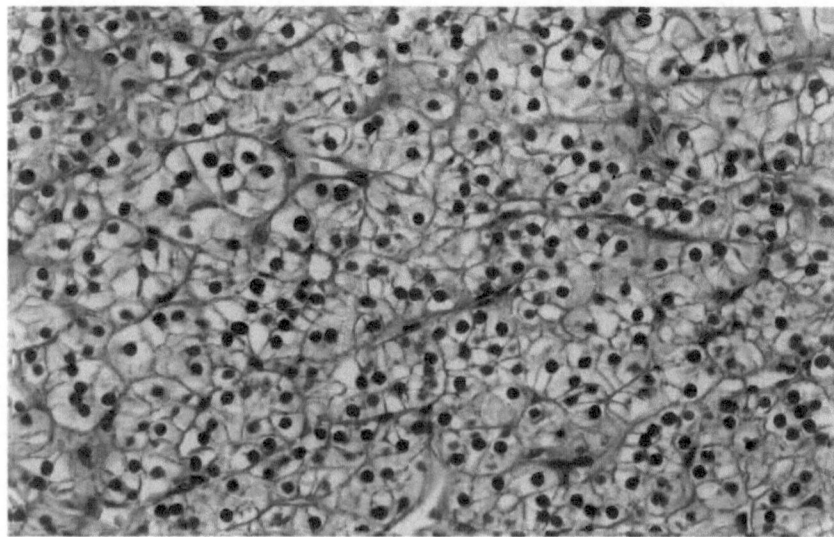

Fig. 92. Primary chief cell hyperplasia (same case as Fig. 91). The encapsulated nodule is composed of chief cells with clear cytoplasm

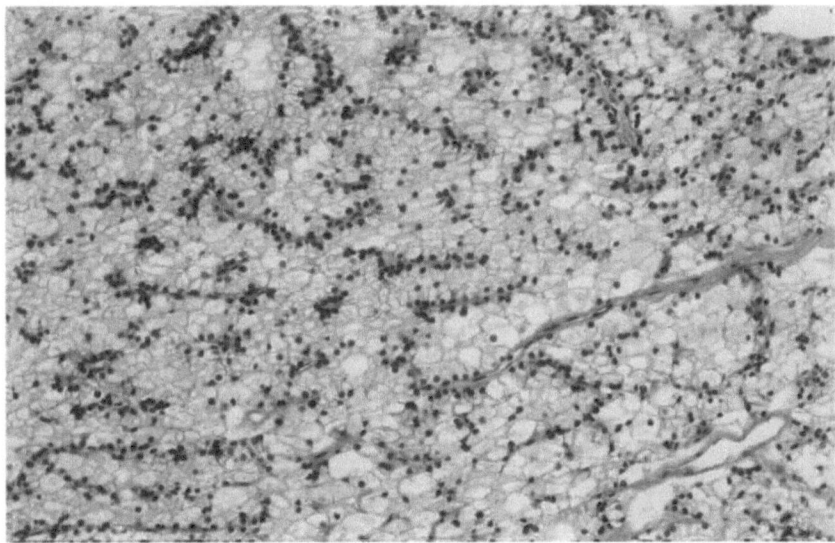

Fig. 93. Primary (water) clear cell hyperplasia. The nuclei of the clear cells are concentrated at the vascular poles of the cells

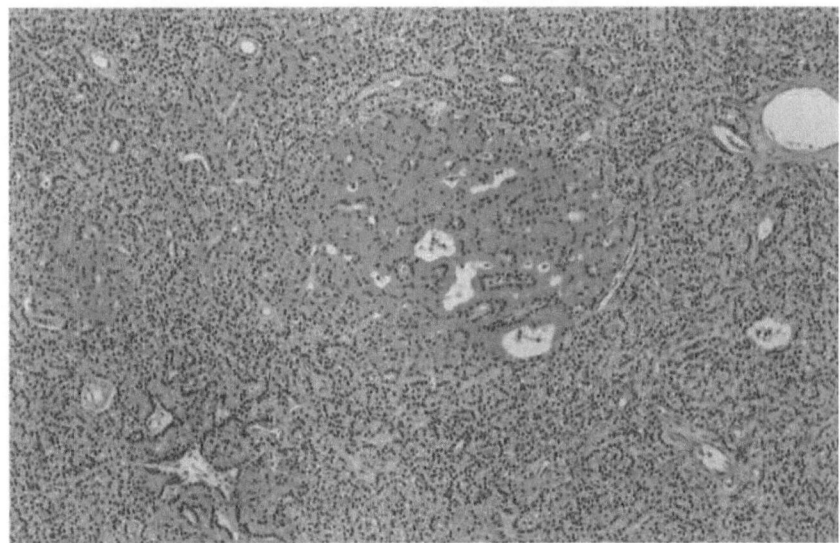

Fig. 94. Hyperplasia associated with secondary hyperparathyroidism. The pattern of hyperplasia is diffuse and nodular

126

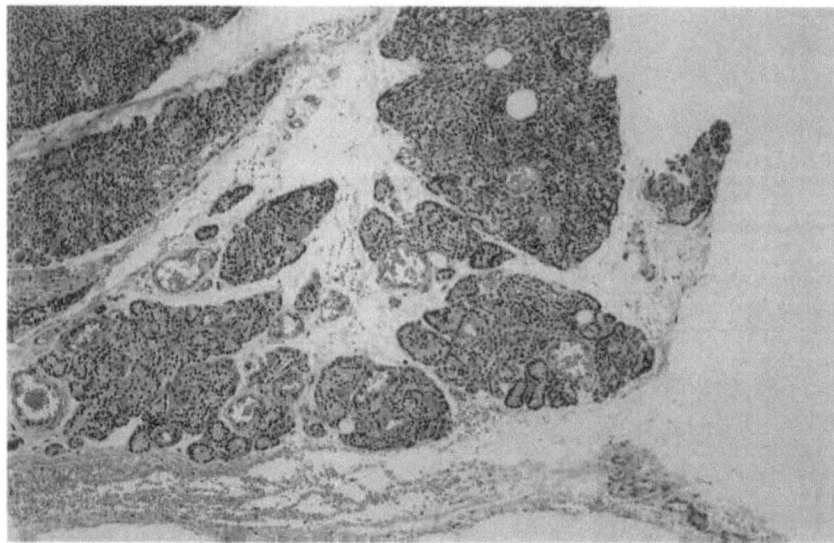

Fig. 95. Parathyromatosis. Clusters of hyperplastic chief cells are present in the soft tissues of the neck in a patient with primary chief cell hyperplasia associated with MEN1

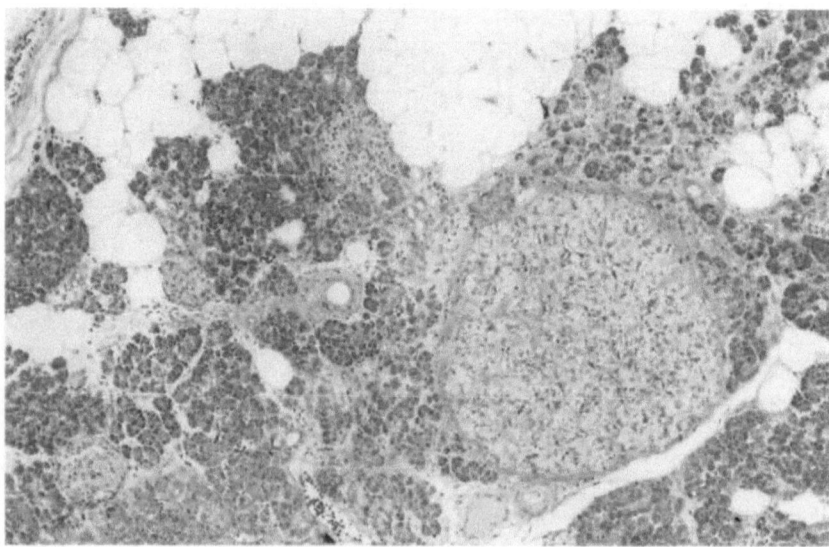

Fig. 96. Well-differentiated endocrine tumour of the pancreas. Microadenoma. All tumour cells were glucagon-immunoreactive in an adjacent section

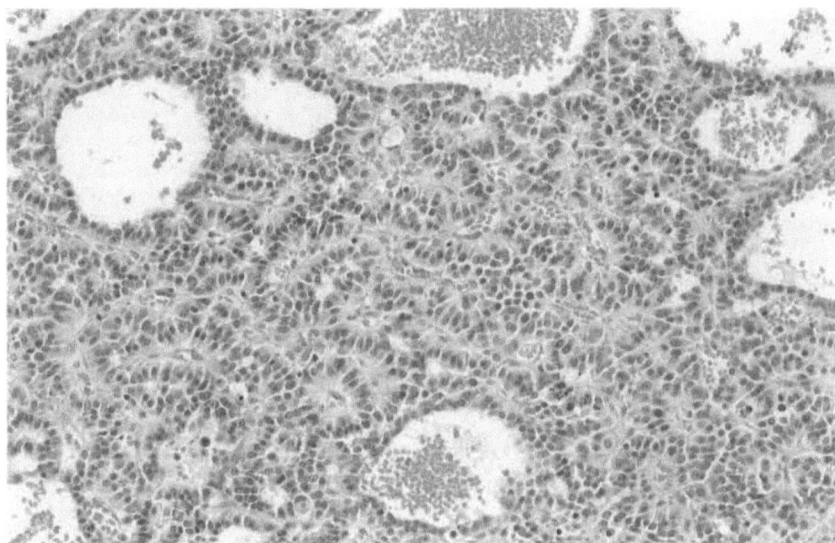

Fig. 97. Well-differentiated endocrine tumour of the pancreas, clinically silent with benign behaviour (macroadenoma). Trabecular pattern

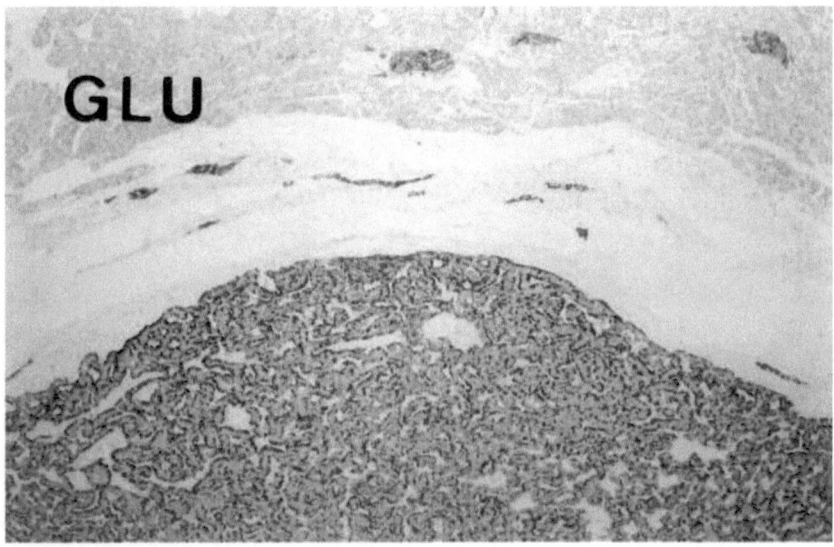

Fig. 98. Well-differentiated endocrine tumour of the pancreas, glucagon producing. Clinically silent and with benign behaviour

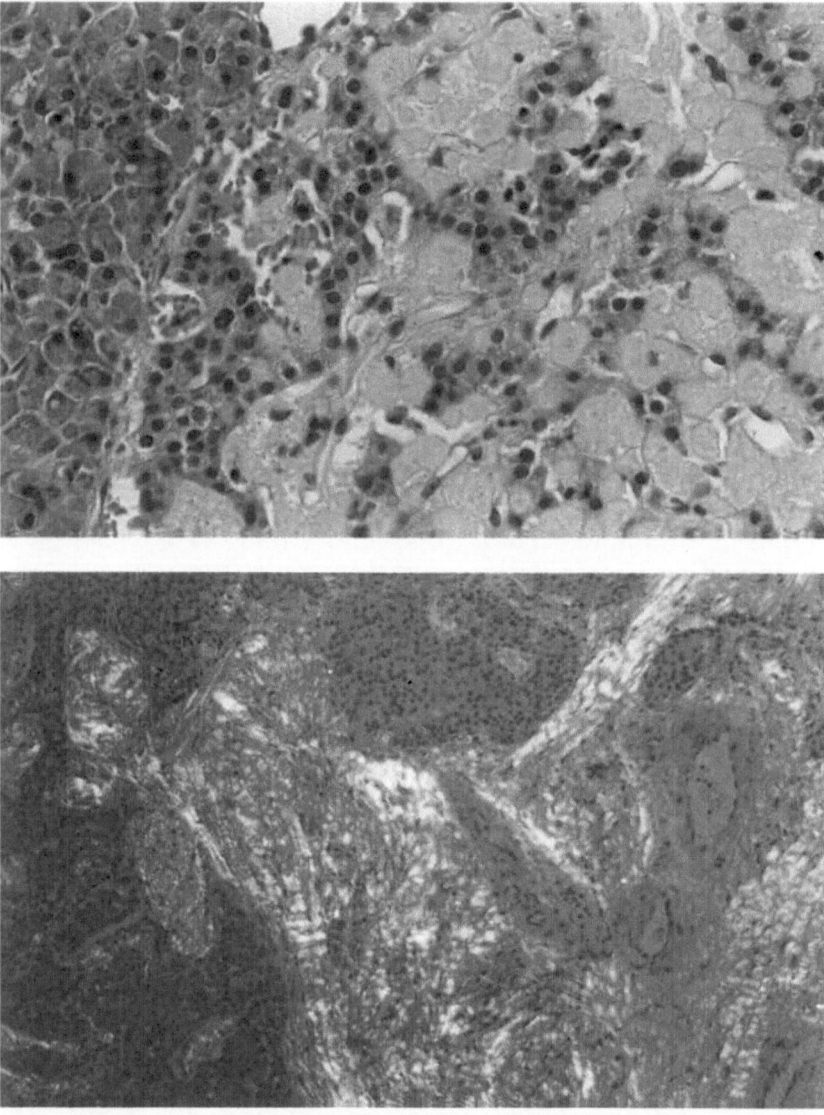

Fig. 99. Well-differentiated endocrine tumour of the pancreas: insulinoma, benign behaviour. *Top* Aggregates of uniform tumour cells are separated by stroma with amyloid deposits. *Bottom* Congo red-haematoxylin stained section showing birefrangent deposits under polarised light

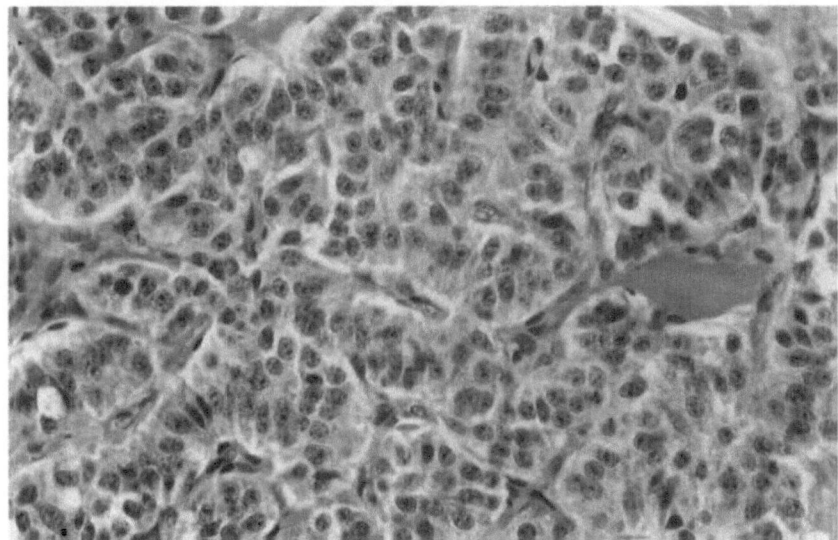

Fig. 100. Well-differentiated endocrine tumour of the pancreas: insulinoma. Uniform tumour cells form trabeculae and small cellular nests separated by scarce vascular stroma. Note a small amyloid deposit

130

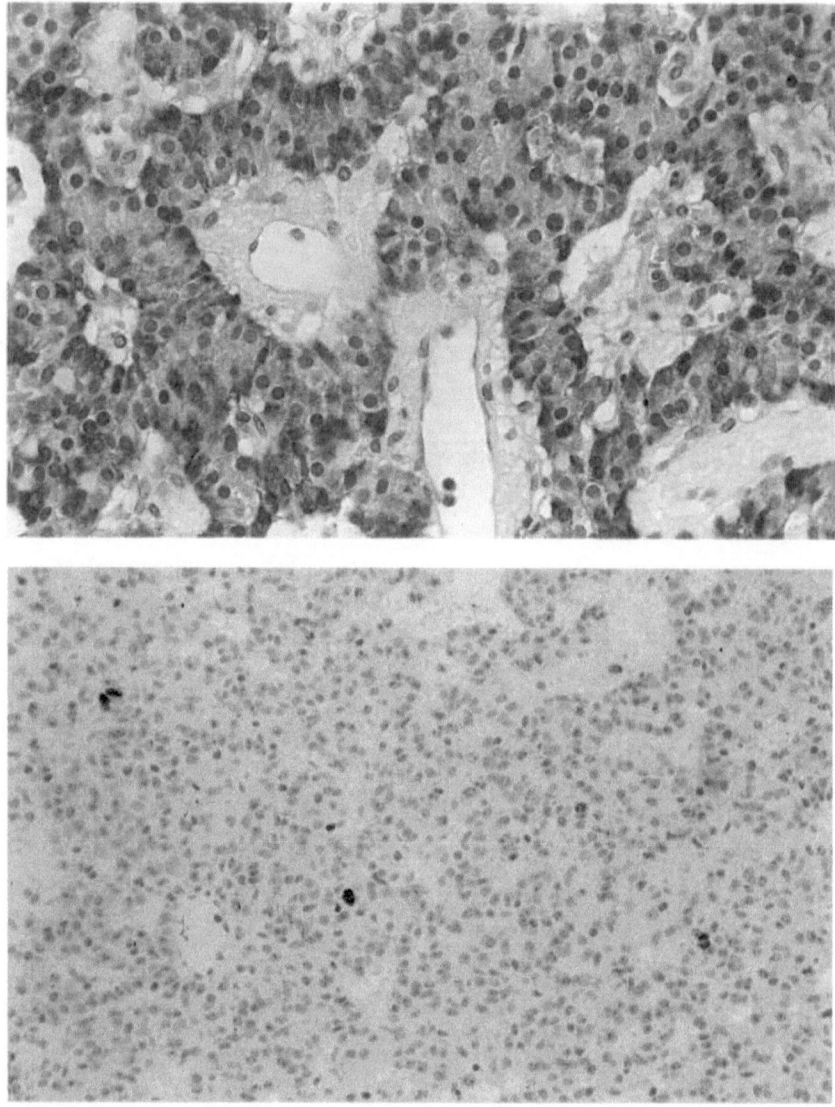

Fig. 101. Well-differentiated endocrine tumour of the pancreas; insulinoma, benign behaviour. *Top* Insulin immunoreactivity of tumour cells forming trabecular aggregates. *Bottom* Scarce Ki67 immunoreactive cells

131

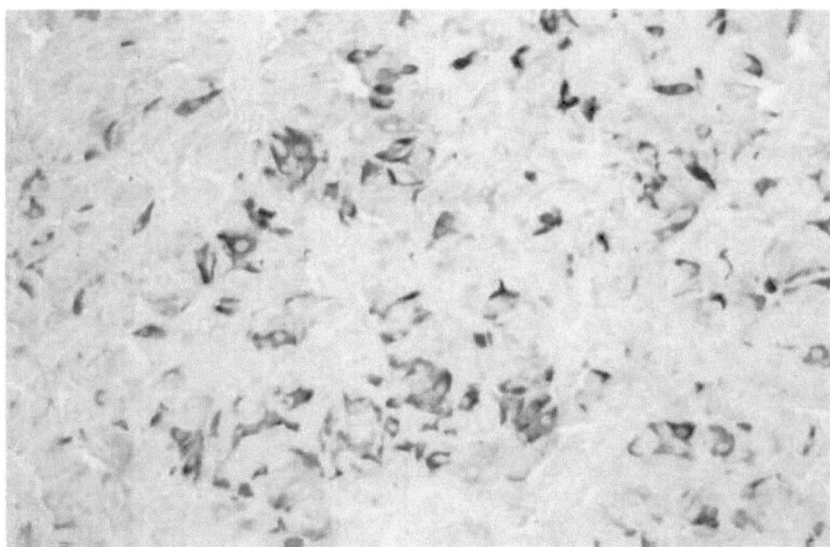

Fig. 102. Well-differentiated endocrine tumour of the pancreas; gastrinoma, uncertain behaviour. Gastrin immunoreactivity of some tumour cells mostly located on the border of trabecular aggregates

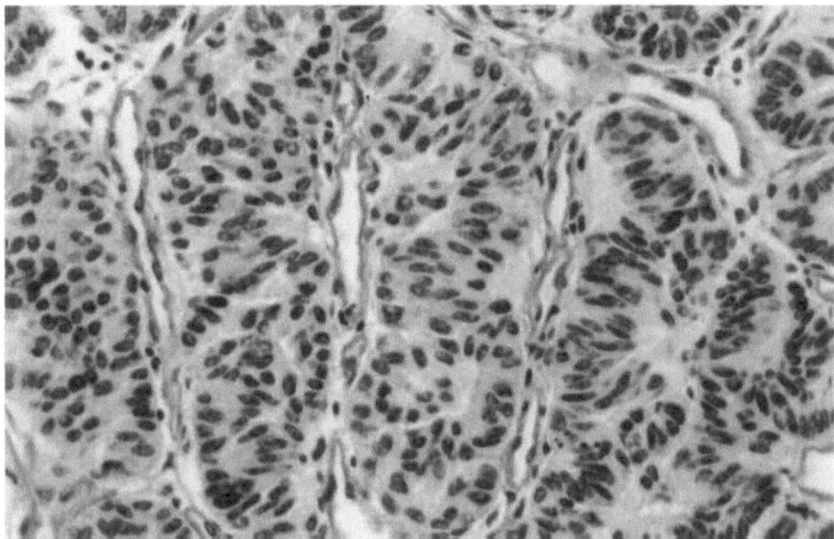

Fig. 103. *Well-differentiated endocrine tumour* of the pancreas; *vipoma*, uncertain behaviour. The tumour cells form gyriform trabeculae. They showed scattered VIP immunoreactivity in adjacent sections

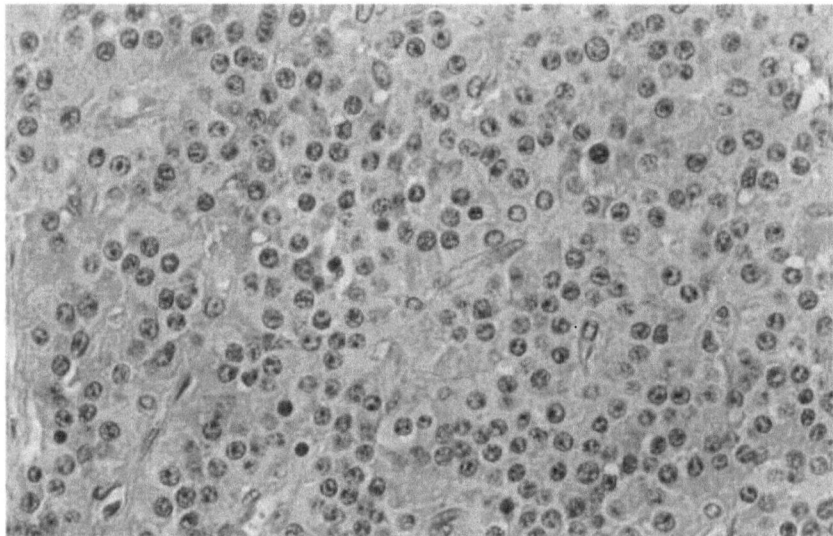

Fig. 104. Well-differentiated endocrine tumour of the pancreas; somatostatinoma, uncertain behaviour. Solid to diffuse aggregates of uniform tumour cells, often with prominent nucleoli; diffuse somatostatin immunoreactivity in adjacent sections

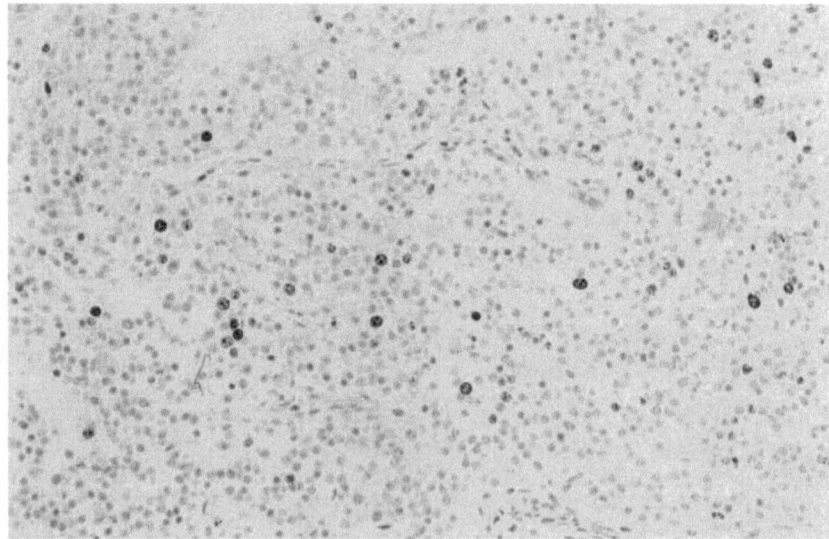

Fig. 105. Well-differentiated endocrine carcinoma of the pancreas; nonfunctioning. Increased (10%) Ki67 immunoreactive cells

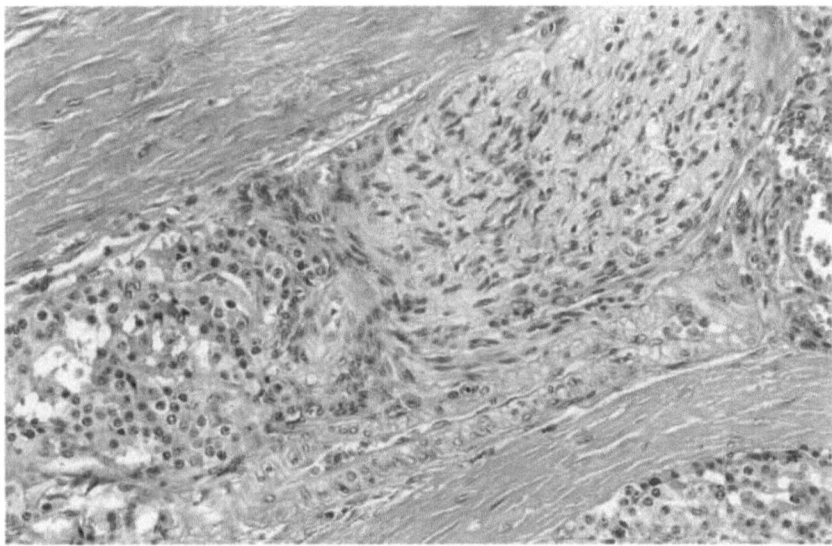

Fig. 106. Well-differentiated endocrine carcinoma of the pancreas; malignant somatostatinoma. Local invasion was found

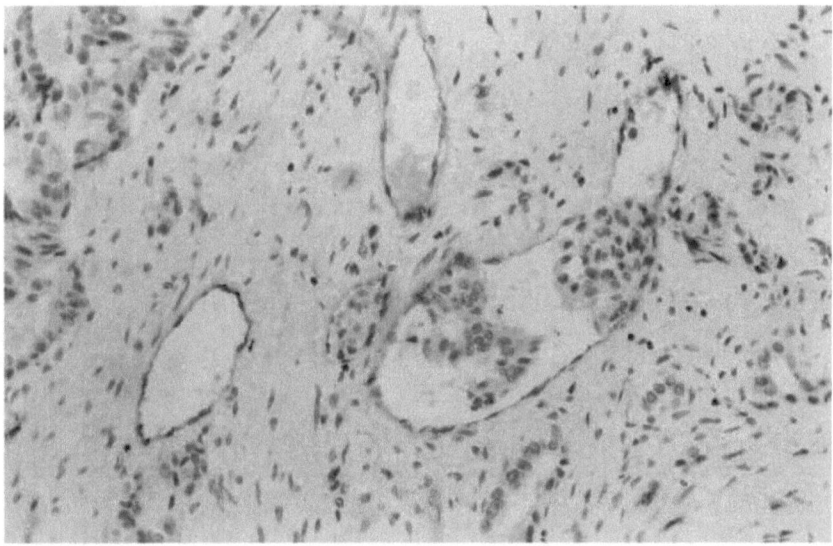

Fig. 107. Well-differentiated endocrine carcinoma of the pancreas; nonfunctioning. Note tumour cell aggregates in peritumour blood vessels stained with Factor VIII antibodies. A liver metastasis was found

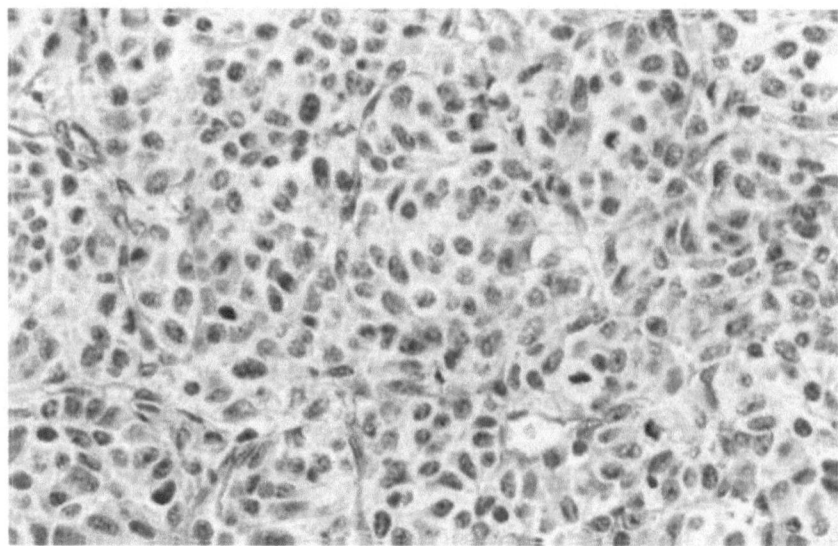

Fig. 108. Well-differentiated endocrine carcinoma of the pancreas; nonfunctioning. Moderate nuclear pleomorphism and increased mitotic rate of tumour cells forming solid aggregates. Invasion of the duodenal wall was found

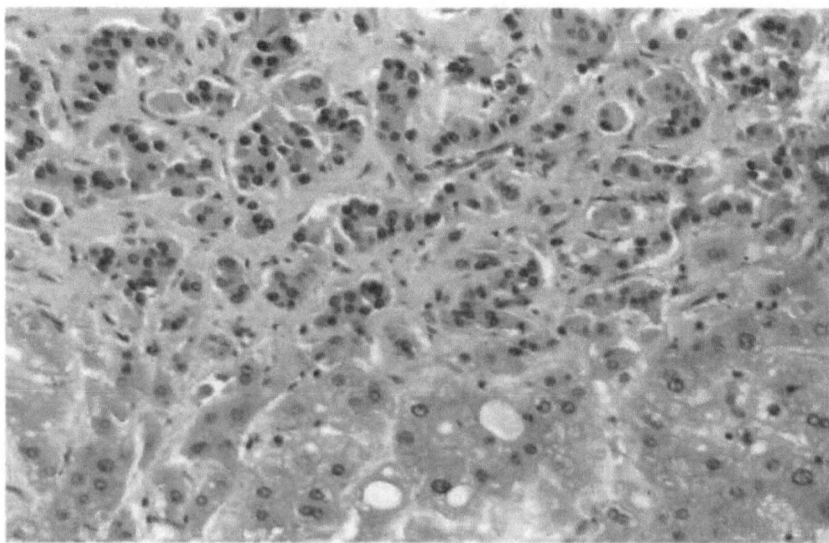

Fig. 109. Well-differentiated endocrine carcinoma of the pancreas; malignant insulinoma. Liver metastasis

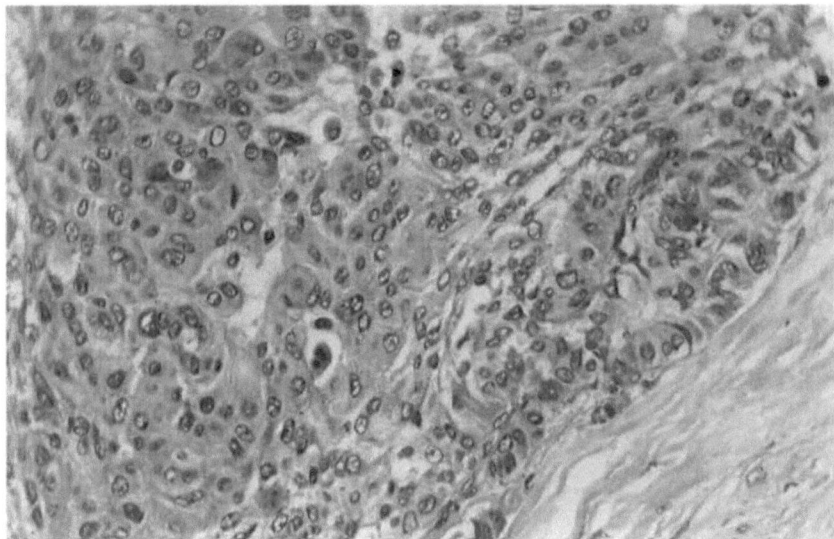

Fig. 110. Well-differentiated endocrine carcinoma of the pancreas; malignant insulinoma. Note nuclear atypia

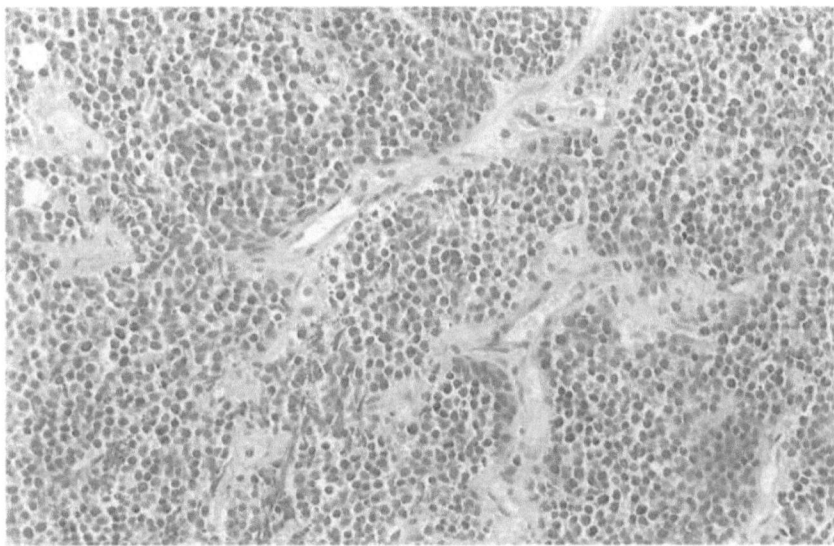

Fig. 111. Poorly differentiated endocrine carcinoma of the pancreas. Solid to diffuse aggregates of small round cells with scarce cytoplasm and relatively large, hyperchromatic, highly atypical nuclei

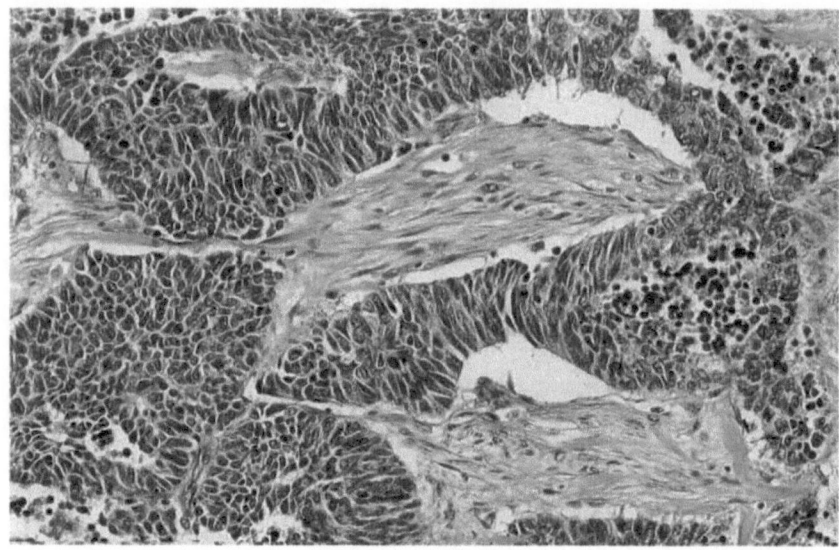

Fig. 112. Poorly differentiated endocrine carcinoma of the pancreas. Solid aggregates of highly atypical spindle to polyhedral cells, with central necrosis and high mitotic index

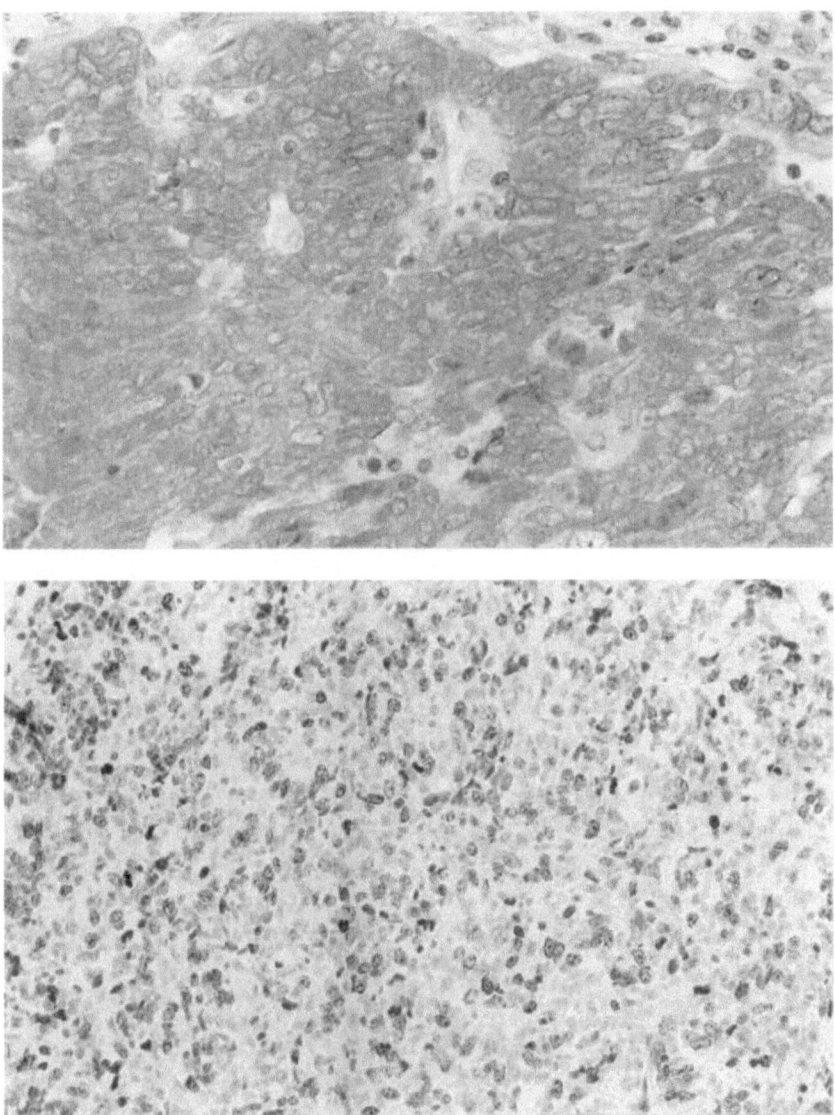

Fig. 113. Poorly differentiated endocrine carcinoma of the pancreas. *Top* Diffuse cytoplasmic immunoreactivity for neuron-specific enolase (NSE). *Bottom* High rate (40%) of Ki67 immunoreactive cells

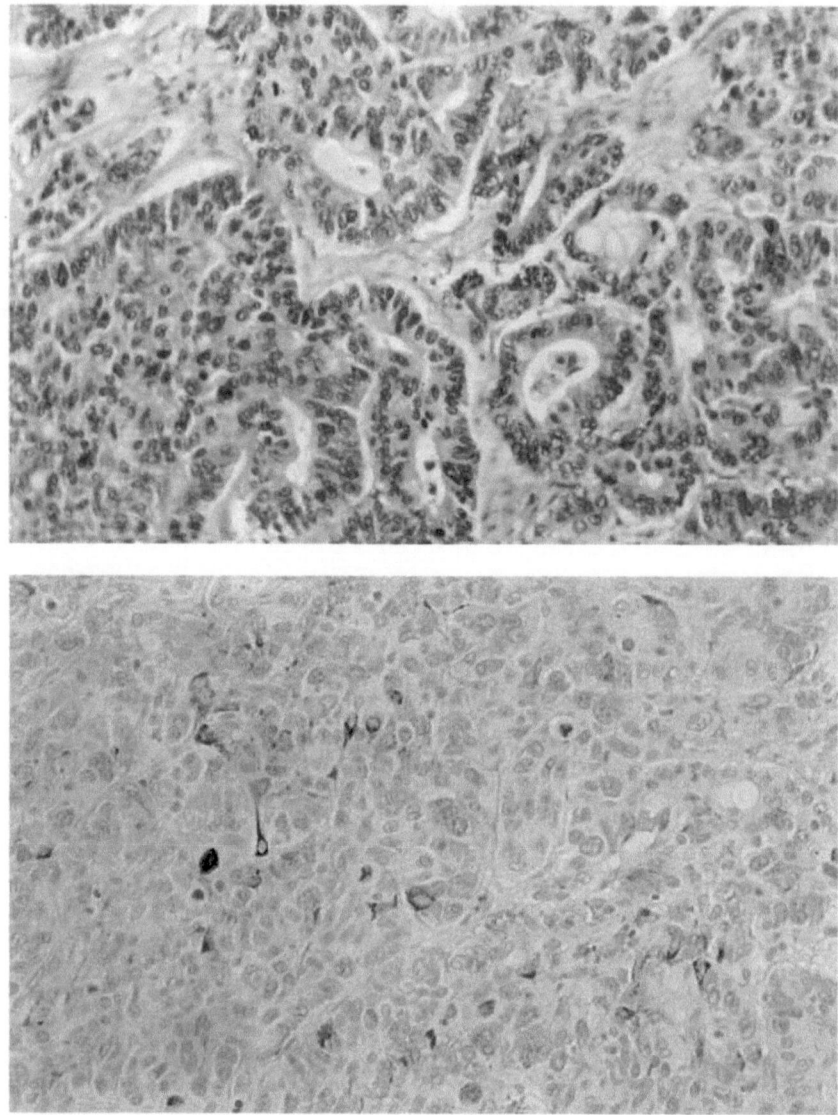

Fig. 114. Mixed exocrine-endocrine carcinoma of the pancreas. *Top* Atypical ductular structure surrounded by cellular aggregates. *Bottom* Immunostain for chromogranin A

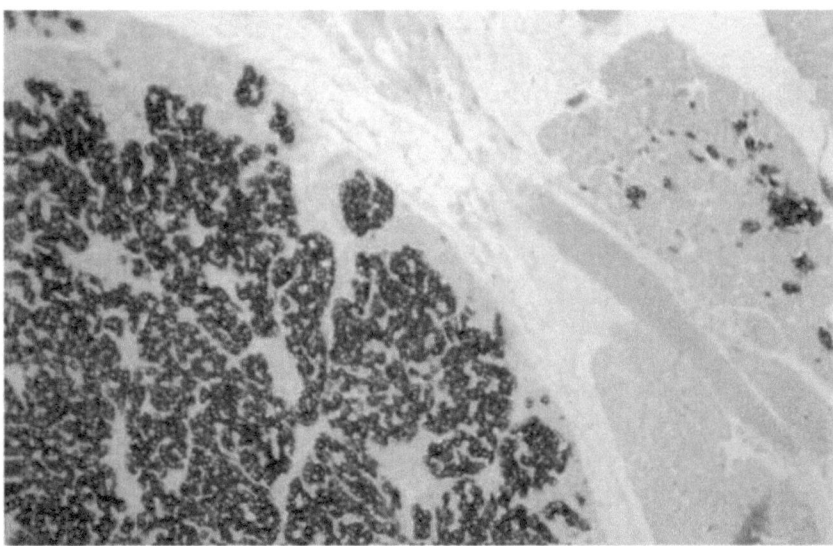

Fig. 115. Neonatal nesidioblastosis, focal. The focus is mainly composed of insulin-immunoreactive cells forming a collection of irregularly sized, shaped, and distributed islet structures

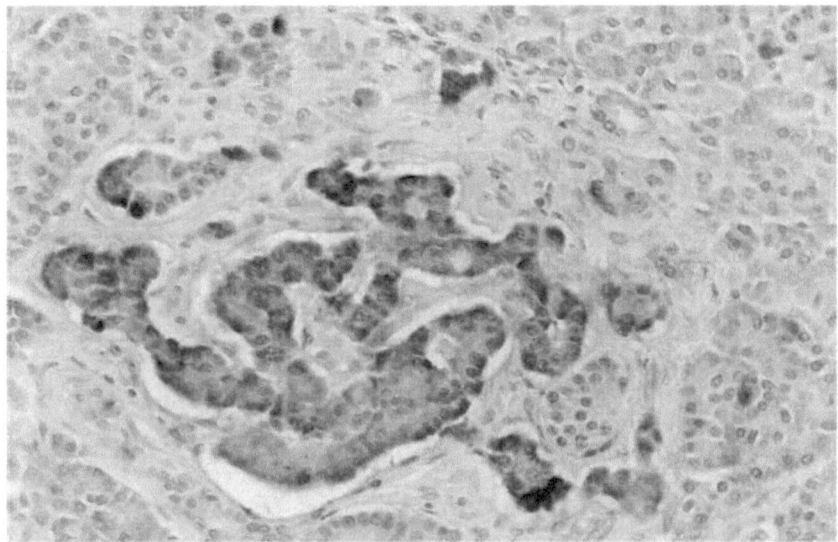

Fig. 116. Islet dysplasia; MEN1 syndrome. Gyriform trabeculae of glucagon-immunoreactive cells replace the islet structure, a remnant of which, glucagon-negative (and insulin positive in an adjacent section), is recognized in the lower right corner

140

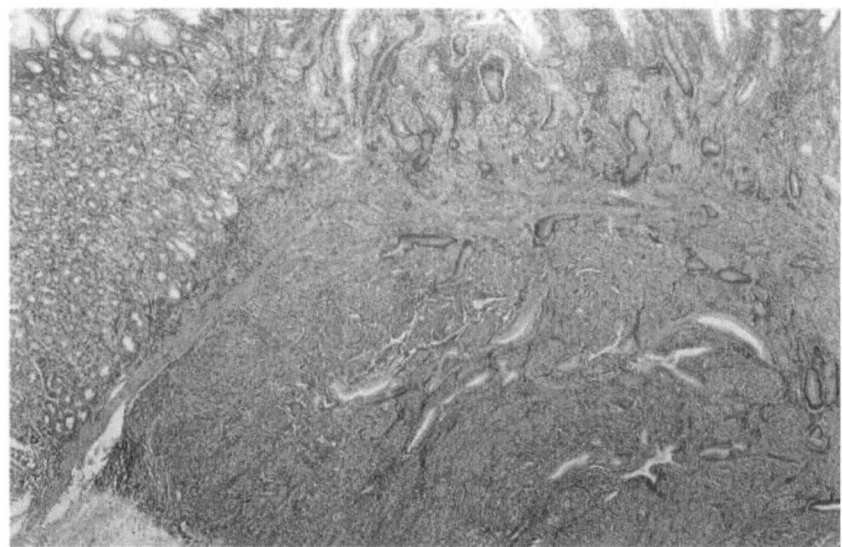

Fig. 117. Well-differentiated endocrine tumour – carcinoid of the stomach, benign behaviour. Mucosal-submucosal ECL cell carcinoid arising in a hypertrophic gastropathy due to MEN1/Zollinger-Ellison syndrome. Note mature, nonatypical glands interspersed with the endocrine growth

Fig. 118. Well-differentiated endocrine tumour – carcinoid of the stomach. *Top* Argyrophil ECL cells form solid nests and trabeculae. Sevier-Munger silver technique. *Bottom* Electron microscopy of vesicular secretory granules, typical of ECL cells ▷

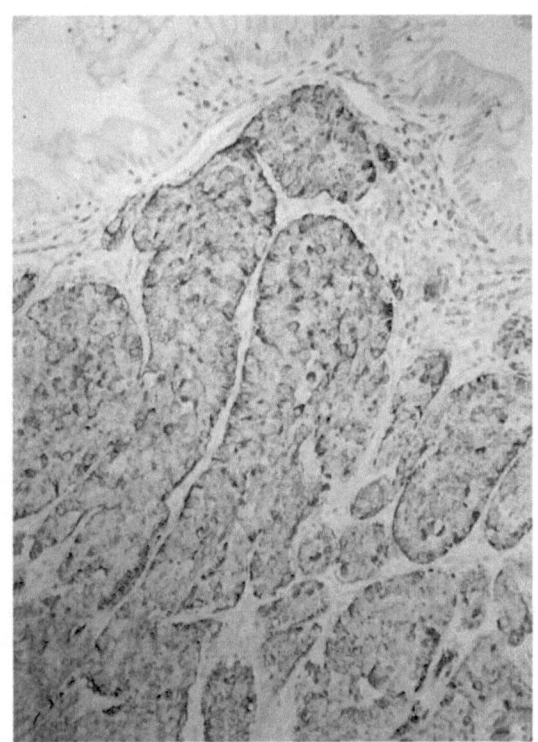

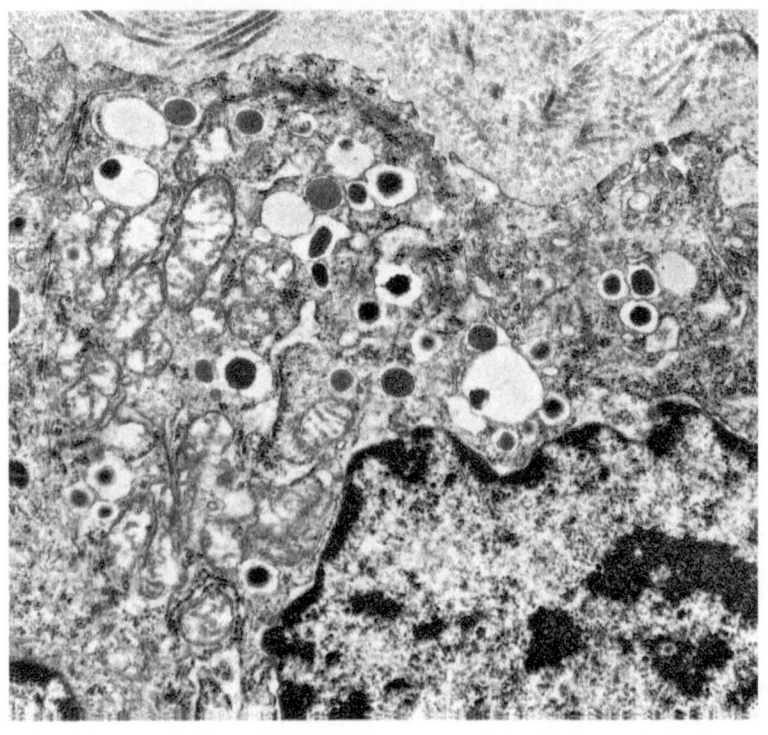

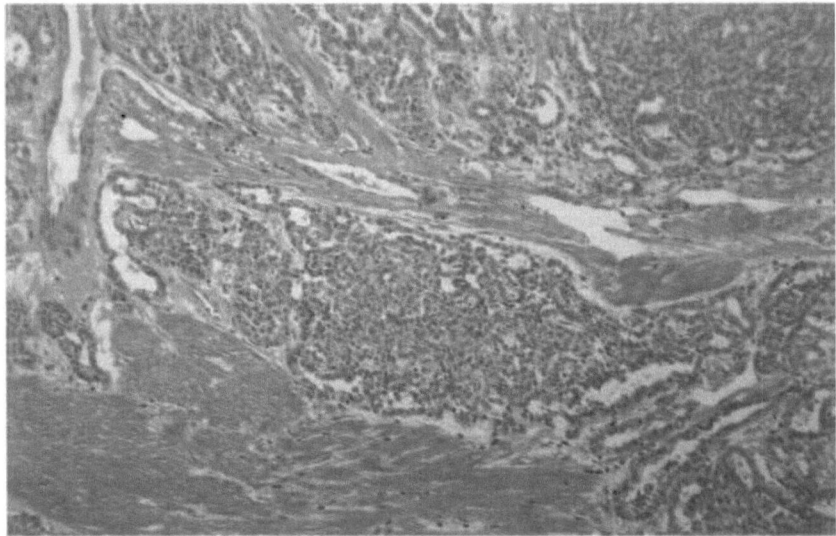

Fig. 119. Well-differentiated endocrine carcinoma – malignant carcinoid of the stomach. Tumour ECL cells in this malignant sporadic carcinoid infiltrate deeply the muscularis propria

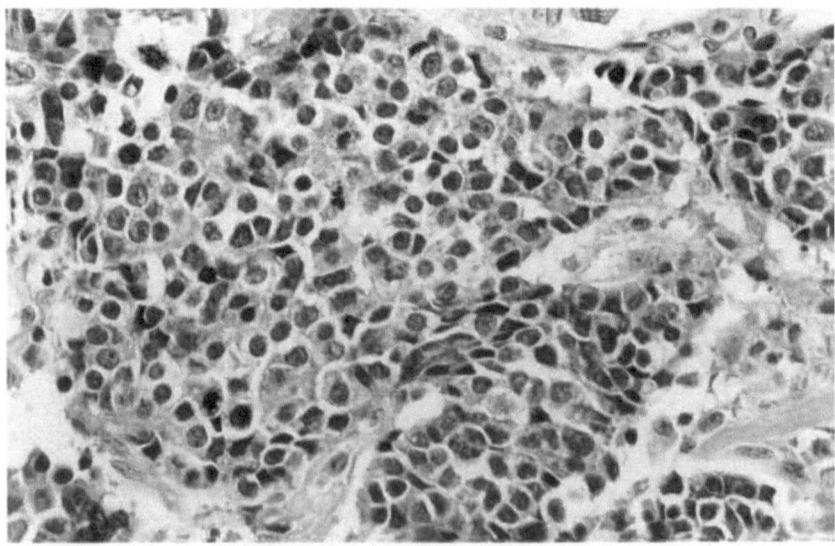

Fig. 120. Poorly differentiated endocrine carcinoma – small cell carcinoma of the stomach. Solid growth of highly atypical cells

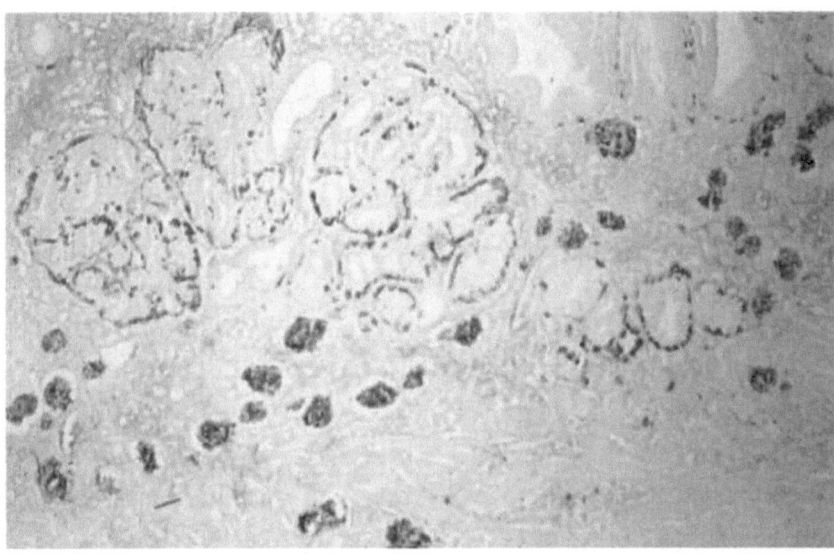

Fig. 121. Endocrine cell hyperplasia in diffuse, corpus-fundus restricted chronic atrophic gastritis (Type A CAG) associated with severe achlorhydria and hypergastrinemia. Grimelius silver shows argyrophil (mostly ECL) cells forming micronodules dispersed in the fibrotic stroma replacing acidopeptic glands and lines at the base of hyperplastic mucous-neck glands

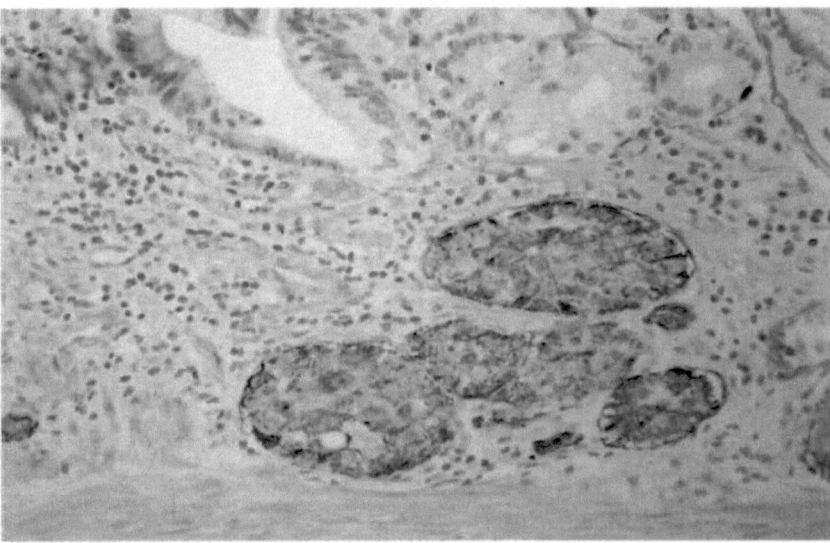

Fig. 122. Endocrine cell dysplasia (precarcinoid lesion) in the corpus mucosa of a MEN1 patient with Zollinger-Ellison syndrome. A collection of enlarged and fused micronodules stained by Sevier-Munger's silver are found deeply in the corpus mucosa

144

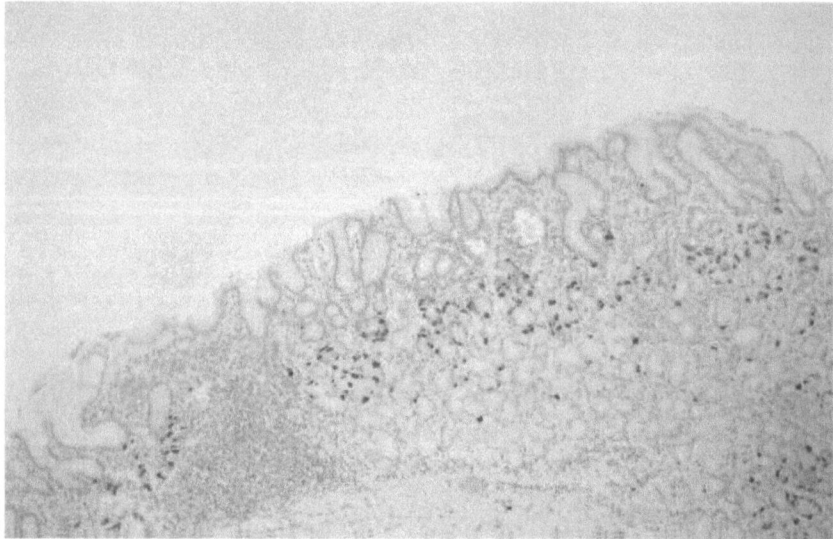

Fig. 123. Gastrin G cell hyperplasia in the pyloric mucosa of an hypergastrinaemic patient with type A CAG and achlorhydria

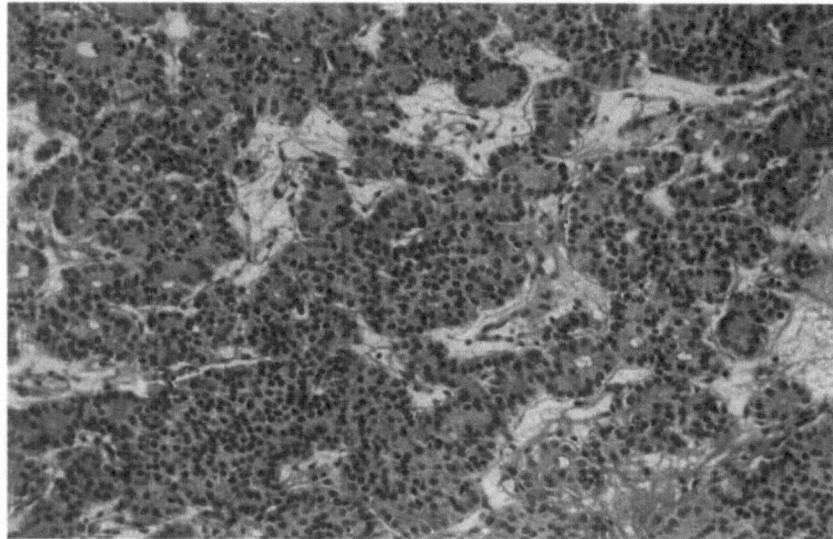

Fig. 124. Well-differentiated endocrine tumour of the duodenum; gastrin-producing, clinically silent, benign behaviour. Uniform tumour cells forming cords and pseudorosettes centred by thin blood vessels

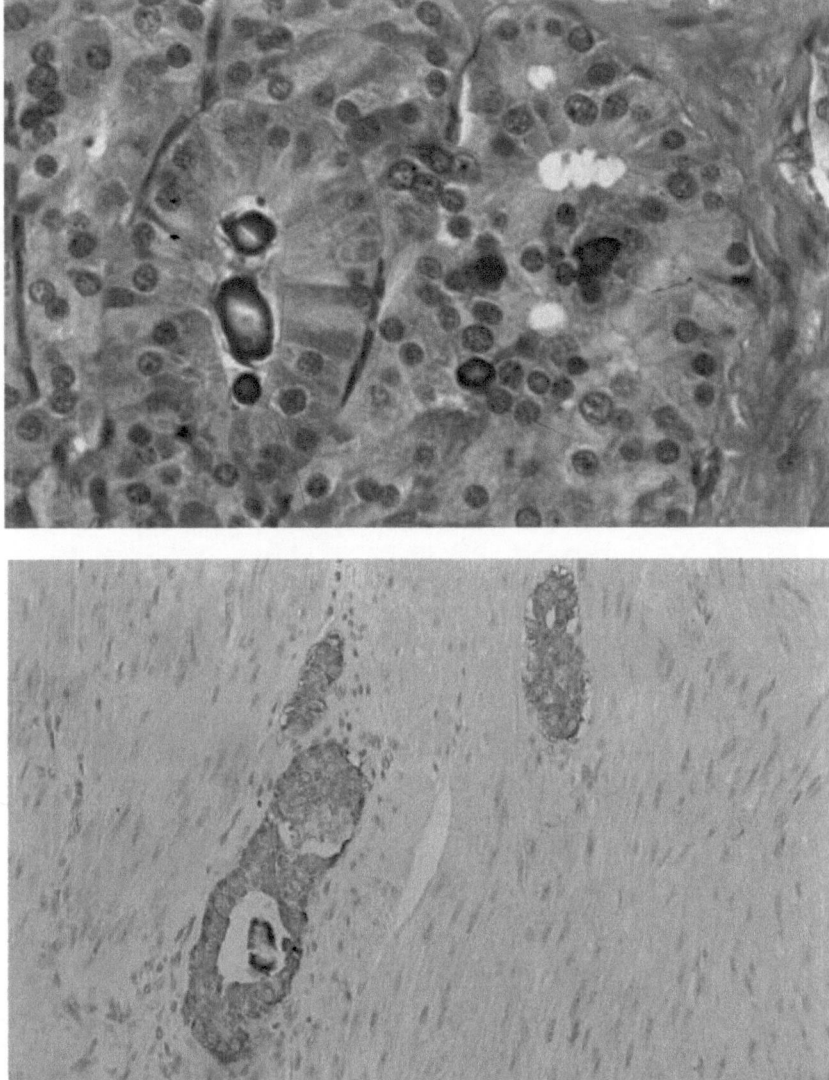

Fig. 125. Well-differentiated endocrine carcinoma of the ampulla; somatostatin-producing. *Top* Tumour cells with abundant cytoplasm form glandular structures with psammoma bodies. *Bottom* Somatostatin immunoreactive tumour nests and glands invade the muscularis propria. Note psammoma-like bodies inside the glands

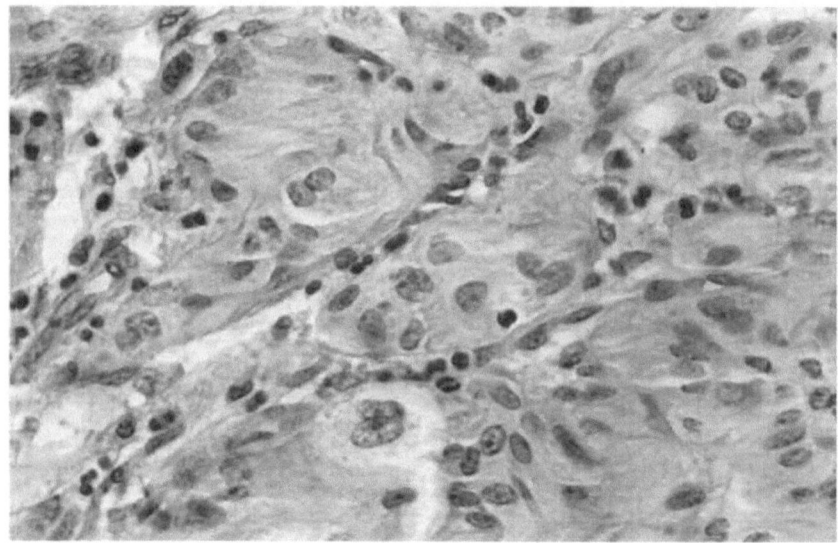

Fig. 126. Gangliocytic paraganglioma of the duodenum, benign behaviour. Epithelial endocrine cell nests are scattered among a neuromatous stroma composed of Schwann-like cells and occasional ganglion cells

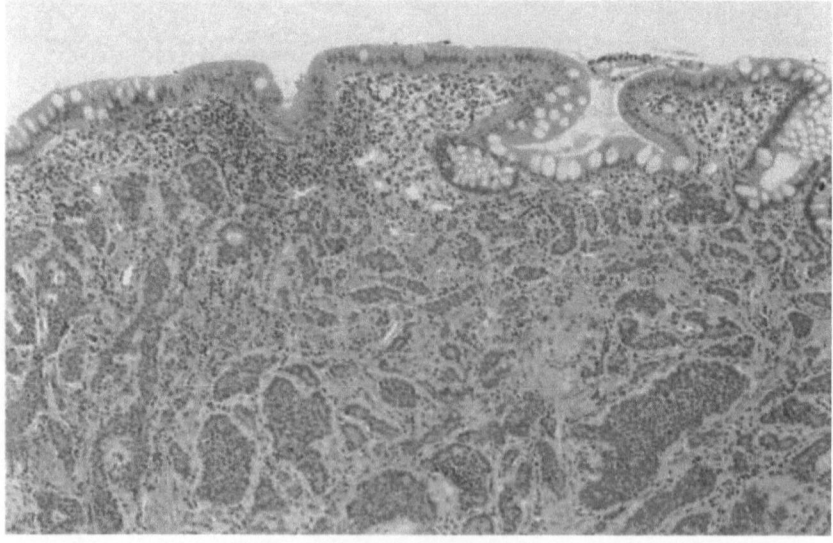

Fig. 127. Well-differentiated serotonin-producing tumour – EC cell carcinoid of the ileum; uncertain behaviour. Tumour cells form solid nests

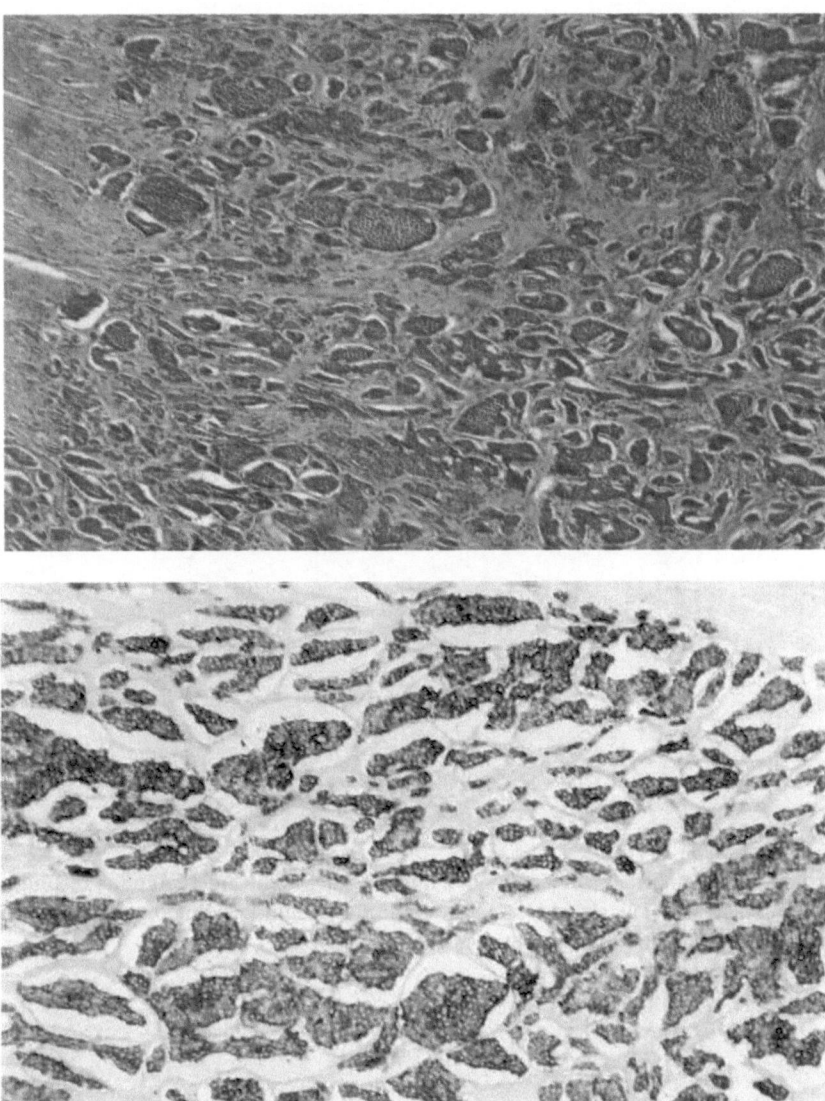

Fig. 128. Well-differentiated serotonin-producing carcinoma – malignant EC cell carcinoid of the ileum, metastatic, with associated carcinoid syndrome. *Top* solid nests with peripheral palisading of tumour cells invade the muscularis propria. *Bottom* Serotonin immunoreactivity of tumour cell nests

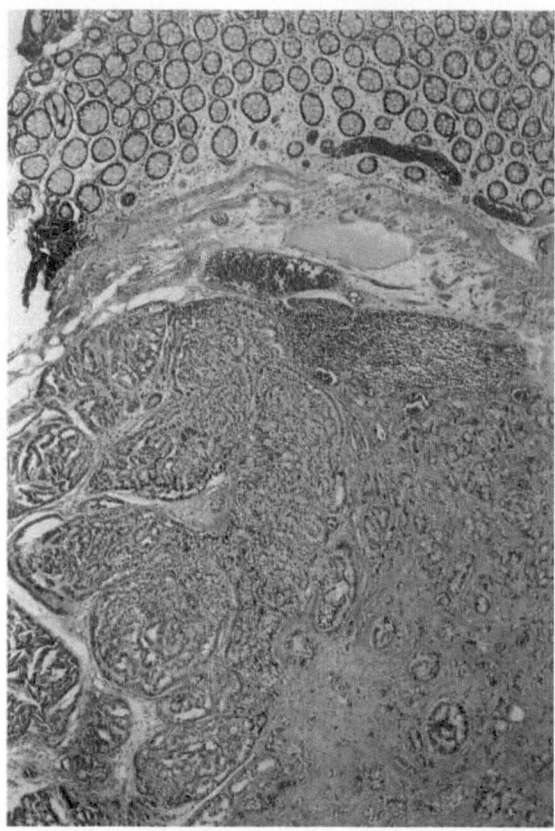

Fig. 129. Well-differentiated endocrine tumour – trabecular carcinoid of the rectum, benign behaviour. The tumour is expanding in the submucosa; enteroglucagon and PP immunoreactivities in adjacent sections

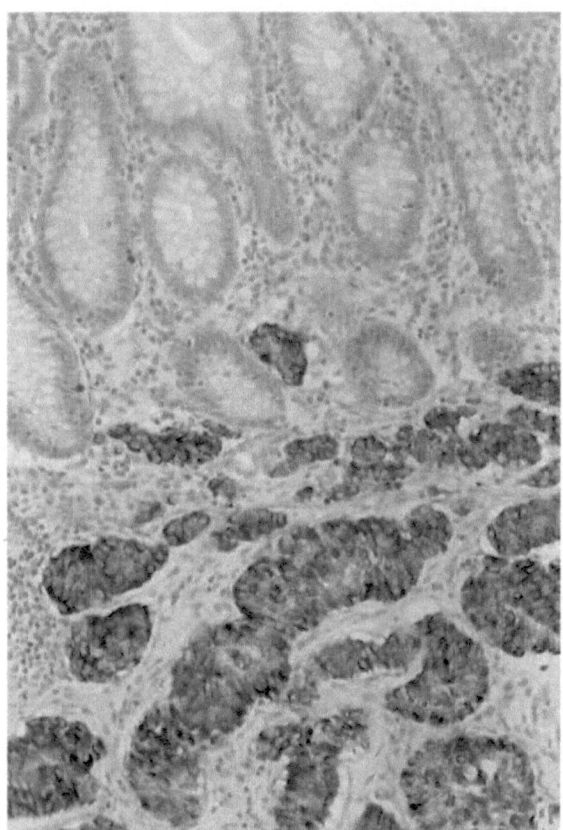

Fig. 130. Well-differentiated endocrine tumour – carcinoid of the appendix, benign behaviour. The tumour is expanding in the submucosa and stains for serotonin

Subject Index